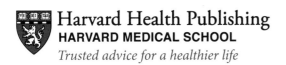

Harvard Health Publishing

HARVARD MEDICAL SCHOOL

*Trusted advice for a healthier life*

Dear Reader,

It's so easy to take your legs for granted. From the time you could walk, they seemed to just be there whenever you needed them—sturdy, reliable limbs that carried you from one place to another without so much as a conscious thought on your part. In fact, you might not recognize just how much you rely on your legs until they hurt or they no longer work as well as they should.

When trouble strikes—if you injure a knee or hip, for example—it quickly becomes clear just how debilitating a leg injury can be. When you can't walk without pain, it can become difficult to work, play sports, exercise, or even climb the stairs from one floor to another in your home. If the damage is significant enough, it can lead to permanent disability. The sheer number of possible conditions that can contribute to leg pain illustrates the need to get medical attention as soon as problems arise. These conditions run the gamut from fractures and sprains to long-term problems caused by vascular disease or diabetes.

Whether you have an acute (short-term) injury such as a ligament tear or a muscle strain from playing sports, or you are experiencing chronic (long-term) knee or hip pain from a condition like arthritis, this report is designed to help you find ways to cope with—and in many cases, resolve—your leg pain. You'll learn where to turn for help and which tests your provider will use to pinpoint your diagnosis. Then, you'll discover the recommended treatments for each type of problem. The solution might be something as simple as rest and over-the-counter pain relievers, or it may involve state-of-the-art surgical procedures and devices. Sometimes a combination of therapies is needed.

Finally, you will learn exercises and other strategies to strengthen your joints and the other structures in your legs, to guard them against injury and disease in the future. It's well worth the effort.

Sincerely,

Robert H. Shmerling, M.D.
*Medical Editor*

Harvard Health Publishing | Harvard Medical School | 4 Blackfan Circle, 4th Floor | Boston, MA 02115

# Why your legs hurt

In theory, your legs should be among the last parts of your body to cause trouble. Tasked with getting you from one place to another, they are among the sturdiest, most powerful features of the human anatomy. In sheer bulk, they account for roughly 40% of your body weight. The thighbone is your largest, strongest bone—so strong, in fact, that it takes approximately 900 pounds of force to break. Similarly, the hip is your largest joint and one of the most stable. And powering it all, the leg and buttock muscles are among the strongest you have. In short, centuries of evolution have prepared your legs to be able to withstand a beating on a daily basis, for decades on end.

Yet there are so many ways for things to go wrong. For example, overweight and obesity can take a toll, adding to stresses on bones, joints, tendons, ligaments, and other tissues. A strong impact—whether from a fall, a sports accident, or a car crash—can cause bones to fracture and muscles to tear. Painful nerve damage can result from a disease such as diabetes or for no identifiable cause. Poor circulation can lead to pain in

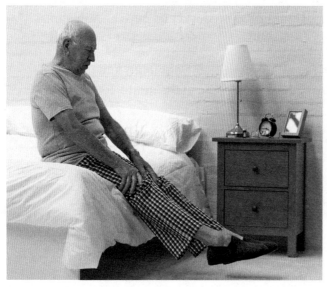

There are so many ways for our legs to develop problems, it's a wonder we don't suffer more leg pain than we do. Fortunately, most of the time, leg trouble does not signal a medical emergency.

the calves and ulcerations of the skin. In fact, there are so many ways for damage to occur, it's a wonder we don't suffer more leg pain than we do.

This report covers more than two dozen of the most common problems to afflict the legs, from arthritis to varicose veins. They are listed in one of four chapters, according to the primary location where they occur—the hip, upper leg, knee, or lower leg. (Note that for the purposes of this report, the legs stop at the ankles. Ankle and foot problems are covered in another Harvard Special Health Report, *Healthy Feet: Preventing and Treating Common Foot Problems*.)

Fortunately, leg problems do not usually signal a medical emergency, but sometimes the condition causing pain can be serious enough to require immediate medical attention (see "When leg pain signals an emergency," page 3). Even if your leg pain does not require urgent action, you should consult a doctor about any persistent, unexplained problem. Sometimes it can signal a systemic problem, such as heart disease or diabetes (see "What your legs tell you about your health," page 5). Even strictly localized problems are worth a visit to the doctor. Medical knowledge about the causes of leg pain has never been greater. There are tests to pinpoint causes that were unclear in the past. And once you have a diagnosis, treatments exist that can at least reduce your pain, if not fully resolve it.

This chapter delves a bit more into why we develop problems with our legs. But first, a broad overview of leg anatomy may be helpful. More detailed anatomical information will follow in each chapter.

## Leg anatomy: An overview

Unlike the hands, which have 27 bones each, or the feet, with 26 apiece, the entire leg has just four bones. Yet the legs are far more complicated than this modest number would imply. To provide the precision you need for running, walking, dancing, jumping, or climbing stairs, each of your legs relies on a complex construction that includes not just bones, but also ligaments, muscles, tendons, nerves, blood vessels, and more.

Bones provide the framework to which the other parts of the leg attach (see Figure 1, page 4). There are three major bones in your legs—the thighbone (femur) in the upper leg, and the shin bone (tibia) and calf bone (fibula) in the lower leg. You may not even be aware of the fibula, but it is a slender bone that runs parallel to the shin bone and helps stabilize it. In addition, the kneecap (patella) is a small bone that protects the knee joint. The bones of the upper and lower legs connect to additional bones in the hips and ankles.

Without the other structures in the leg, however, bones would collapse into a useless heap. Specifically:

- Ligaments are the tough bands of connective tissue that connect bones to other bones. They link the thighbone and shin bone at the knee joint and connect the thighbone to the pelvis at the hip joint. Ligaments also stabilize joints, restricting movement to a range that will not cause damage. (For a more detailed discussion, see "Hip anatomy 101," page 7, and "Knee anatomy 101," page 27.)
- Muscles provide the force to move bones at the joints. In the upper leg, these include the powerful quadriceps muscles on the front of the thigh, the hamstrings at the back of the thigh, and the hip flexors (most notably, the iliopsoas), which help you lift your thigh. In the calf, the gastrocnemius

## When leg pain signals an emergency

Most leg pain results from gradual wear and tear or minor issues that will resolve in time or with conservative treatment. Yet, a few symptoms signal a much more serious problem that requires immediate attention. Call a doctor or 911 or go to an emergency room if you think you might have one of these conditions.

**Avascular necrosis.** Certain diseases, such as sickle cell anemia, or an injury such as a fracture or dislocation can damage the vessels that supply blood to bones in the leg. Also called osteonecrosis, avascular necrosis occurs when a disruption in the blood supply causes the bone to die. Eventually, the bone can break apart and collapse.

*Symptoms:* Bone pain, which may begin suddenly and increases over time.

**Bone cancer.** Bone cancer is rare, accounting for less than 1% of all cancers. Most cancer in the bones has traveled there from other organs, such as from the breast or prostate gland. Cancer can damage and weaken bone to the point where it fractures.

*Symptoms:* Bone pain, fatigue, unintended weight loss, swelling in the area, fractures, especially in someone with a prior diagnosis of cancer.

**Compartment syndrome.** In this serious condition, pressure within the muscles and other tissues in the legs builds to the point where it prevents oxygen-rich blood from reaching nerves and muscles. Without treatment, it can lead to permanent muscle and nerve damage.

*Symptoms:* Intense pain, a feeling of tightness or fullness in the affected muscle, tingling or burning.

**Deep-vein thrombosis (DVT).** DVT is a blood clot that forms in a deep vein of the leg (see "Deep-vein thrombosis," page 17). It can occur when blood flow slows—for example, after surgery, or when you've been immobile for many hours on a long car or plane trip. If the clot travels to a lung and becomes lodged there, it's called a pulmonary embolism—a life-threatening condition.

*Symptoms:* Swelling and redness in the leg, tenderness. If the clot travels to the lung, symptoms may include shortness of breath, chest pain, and coughing.

**Arterial thrombosis.** This occurs when a blood clot forms in an artery. If the clot is not treated, the condition may lead to gangrene (with a dark discoloration of the toes or foot).

*Symptoms:* Sudden pain and swelling in one leg, accompanied by discoloration.

**Fracture.** The force of an accident or weakening due to osteoporosis or cancer can cause a bone to fracture, or break. Fractures range in severity from a simple break in one bone to a shattering in which a bone breaks into multiple pieces or pierces the skin.

*Symptoms:* Pain, swelling and tenderness of the skin over the injury, bruising, deformity, trouble moving or using the injured leg.

and soleus muscles help you point and flex your foot, walk, jump, and run. The gluteus maximus, medius, and minimus muscles of the buttocks give shape to your rear end, support your lower body, and allow your hips to rotate.

- Tendons are the strong bands of connective tissue that attach muscles to bones. One of the best-

## Figure 1: Anatomy of the legs

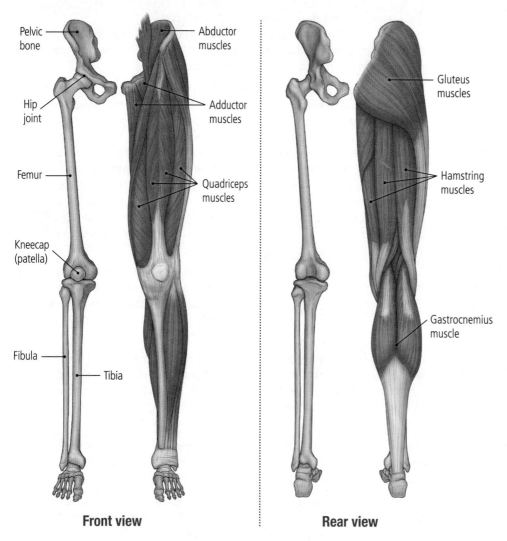

Pelvic bone

Hip joint

Femur

Kneecap (patella)

Fibula

Tibia

Abductor muscles

Adductor muscles

Quadriceps muscles

**Front view**

Gluteus muscles

Hamstring muscles

Gastrocnemius muscle

**Rear view**

The femur is the main bone of the upper leg, while the fibula and tibia bones make up the lower leg. The patella protects the knee. Thick, strong quadriceps muscles cover the front of the upper thigh. In the back of the leg are the hamstrings and gastrocnemius muscles.

known tendons in the body is the Achilles tendon, which connects your calf muscle to your heel.

However, producing movement takes more than having all the anatomical parts strung together, like a skeleton in a biology lab. To move smoothly, groups of muscles must flex and extend, contract and relax in complementary fashion. Otherwise you would move in a stiff, awkward, or jerky manner, like Frankenstein.

To guide their movements, muscles receive instructions from the brain, which sends its messages using electrical signals that travel through nerves. Motor nerves tell you which muscles to flex and relax. But signals also travel back up to the brain from your legs and feet. Sensory nerves tell you where your leg and foot are in space. They tell you where the ground is, whether it's slippery or uneven, and where there's a pebble so you don't step too hard. Temperature receptors can alert you to something that's dangerously hot or cold, while pressure receptors are sensitive to compression and tell you whether something is touching your leg or foot.

In order to bend, straighten, and support the body's weight, the legs also rely on a steady supply of oxygen- and nutrient-rich blood pumped from the heart. A network of arteries delivers blood from the heart to the legs. Another network of blood vessels, the veins, ferries oxygen-depleted blood back to the heart and lungs.

The circulatory system is a finely tuned hydraulic masterpiece. If it weren't, how could it force blood to flow upward, against gravity? If gravity alone ruled, all of your blood would soon pool in your feet. To keep the blood moving, your veins contain tiny valves that close as the blood passes through, preventing it from flowing backward. In addition, as you walk or run, your calf muscles compress and relax, helping to squeeze the blood back up.

## Who gets leg pain?

Any of the structures in the legs can develop problems, so perhaps it's not surprising that virtually all of us suffer leg pain at some point. Leg pain can strike at any age. In childhood, you may have had growing pains or broken a leg. As an adult, you're more likely to suffer muscles strains or shin splints. In advanced age, arthritis becomes increasingly likely. According to the CDC, nearly half of Americans have knee osteoarthritis by age 85, and a quarter develop hip osteoarthritis.

The vulnerability of the legs comes in part from the fact that we rely on these limbs for so much. While it's true the legs are designed for durability, the human life span for most of evolutionary time was much shorter than it is today. For millennia, people commonly lived only 30 to 40 years. Legs didn't have to last longer than that.

Your joints are particularly vulnerable because of their complexity and the stresses you subject them to. Your knees and hips are your largest joints. While supporting your weight as you stand upright, they must also execute the complex maneuvers involved in a broad variety of movements. For example, getting in and out of a car may seem simple when the hips and knees are fine, but if you have hip arthritis or torn cartilage in your knee, the amount of flexing, turning, and balancing required by these maneuvers can be quite challenging. So it's not surprising, given all that your knees and hips do, that they're prone to injuries and deterioration. That's why nearly half of this report relates to knees and hips.

But problems can also develop in muscles, nerves, or blood vessels. Poor circulation in the arteries can produce calf pain (claudication; see "Peripheral artery disease and claudication," page 43), and people with diabetes can have blood flow problems that lead to skin ulcers. Veins, too, can cause trouble if the little valves in the veins no longer function properly. This condition, known as venous insufficiency,

causes fluid to pool in your lower extremities—a problem known medically as edema (see page 41).

## What your legs tell you about your health

The primary purpose of your legs is to keep you upright and mobile. Yet, your legs can also act as an indicator of your overall health. Although some symptoms you may experience are specific to a leg problem, others can suggest trouble with your heart, nervous system, kidneys, or other organs. Use the following symptom guide to help you decipher what broader problems your leg pain might suggest.

**Symptom: Leg cramps.**

**Possible cause: Dehydration.** A cramp in your leg after you've been working out, especially in the heat, could be an important sign that your body is low on fluids. To contract and relax normally, muscles rely on water and electrolytes like sodium and potassium. Too little fluid or electrolytes can hypersensitize the nerves that control muscles in the legs, causing the muscles to contract abnormally, or spasm.

All of your organs rely on fluids to function normally. Dehydration prevents cells from properly using energy, transporting nutrients, and dividing. If not quickly remedied, it can become a life-threatening condition. To avoid getting too low on fluids, drink water or an electrolyte-containing sports drink before, during, and after exercise.

**Symptom: Calf pain during activity.**

**Possible cause: Atherosclerosis.** Pain in your legs that's triggered by activity—along with weak pulses in your legs and feet, pale skin, and sores on your legs or feet that don't heal well—are signs of peripheral artery disease (see page 43), a blockage in blood flow to your legs. The most likely cause is atherosclerosis, a

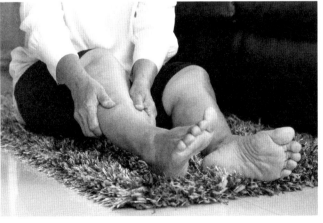

Poor circulation in the arteries (peripheral artery disease) can produce a type of calf pain known as claudication. By contrast, leg cramps after you work out are likely the result of dehydration.

hardening and narrowing of the arteries as a result of sticky cholesterol and fat deposits called plaques.

If your legs are suffering from inadequate blood flow, likely your heart is, too. Peripheral artery disease shares risk factors with heart disease—namely, smoking, high cholesterol, diabetes, and high blood pressure. It increases your risk of developing heart disease and of having a heart attack or stroke in the future. Peripheral artery disease is a serious condition. To avoid complications, you need to make changes to your lifestyle by losing excess weight, getting more active, eating a heart-healthy diet, and quitting smoking. Sometimes surgery is needed to open up or bypass a blocked artery. Your doctor may recommend blood thinners and vasodilators (medications that help open up blood vessels).

**Symptoms: Pain, burning, numbness, and tingling.**

**Possible cause: Diabetes.** These feelings in your legs or feet could be signs of diabetic neuropathy—nerve damage due to persistently high blood sugar (see "Peripheral neuropathy," page 45). High blood sugar damages not only the small blood vessels that send oxygen and nutrients to the nerves, but also the nerves themselves, preventing them from sending the correct signals to your brain.

The keys to preventing neuropathy, as well as other diabetes complications like vision loss, heart disease, and kidney damage, are to keep your blood sugar under good control and modify other risk factors. Don't smoke; also, bring down high blood pressure and cholesterol. Tight blood sugar control requires a combination of dietary changes, physical activity, blood sugar monitoring, and sometimes blood sugar–lowering medications.

**Symptom: Leg swelling.**

**Possible causes: Heart, kidney, or liver disease.** Many things can cause swelling in the legs. At the least worrisome level, it may be the result of an injury, such as a sprain or strain, or venous insufficiency (see "Edema," page 41). Or it could point to a more serious problem, such as

- a blood clot in the leg (see "Deep-vein thrombosis," page 17)
- heart failure
- kidney disease or kidney failure
- liver disease (cirrhosis).

Each of these conditions is unique and requires you to work with your doctor to get a diagnosis and start on a treatment plan.

**Symptom: Slow walking (in older adults).**

**Possible cause: Problems with multiple organ systems.** If you've ever watched a parent or grandparent slow down with age, you know how concerning this sign can be. Research suggests that your walking speed may be a marker for your overall health, to the point where the pace at which you walk may be able to predict your life expectancy. In one study published in *JAMA*—a pooled analysis of nine studies with a total of 34,000 participants, ages 65 and older—walking speed was just as good a predictor of life expectancy as a host of other health indicators, such as chronic conditions, smoking history, blood pressure, body mass index, and hospitalizations. Across the entire range of gait speeds—parsed by as little as inches per second—those who walked faster lived longer.

Walking relies on multiple organ systems working well and in tandem—the circulatory system, nervous system, musculoskeletal system, and nervous system. A slowed gait could indicate a problem with one or more of these systems. One day, doctors might use walking speed to evaluate your health, just as they currently use electrocardiograms and blood pressure measurements. Until then, keep a watchful eye on your walking speed. ♥

# Hip pain

Watch a ballet dancer, and you can appreciate the hip joint's ability to move in almost any direction, if only the muscles are willing. The hip is a ball-and-socket joint with a remarkable range of motion. It is also both the largest and sturdiest joint in the body. With a protective girdle of strong muscles surrounding it, the hip joint was built for endurance.

It isn't indestructible, however. Osteoarthritis is one of the leading causes of chronic hip pain, especially as you age. If a fall or another injury leads to intense pain, you could have a fracture. Pain on the outside of your hip or thigh suggests an issue with the muscles, ligaments, or tendons.

This chapter contains an overview of some of the most common problems that can cause hip pain (listed in alphabetical order), along with a description of treatments that are available. It starts with a review of hip anatomy, to familiarize you with the various structures you will be reading about in this chapter.

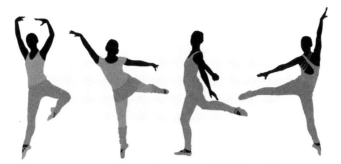

The hip—the largest and sturdiest joint in the body—allows a remarkable range of motion, and it can take a pounding for decades. But over time, osteoarthritis and other problems can develop.

*© Getty Images*

## Hip anatomy 101

As the old song says, "The hip bone's connected to the thighbone." But that simple line doesn't do justice to the complicated, finely tuned machinery of the hip's ball-and-socket joint. To support the full weight of your body while allowing movement in different directions, the top of the thighbone is shaped as a smooth ball that fits snugly within the socket of the pelvis. In addition to the bones themselves, muscles, ligaments, cartilage, and bursae all play important roles. While people tend to think of the hip as a single bone they can feel on the side of the body, the hip is actually a large region that extends to the groin and thigh.

### Bones

Key bone structures in the hip include

- the ilium (the uppermost and largest part of the pelvis; see Figure 2, page 8)
- the femur (thighbone)
- the femoral head (the rounded top of the thighbone, which serves as the ball of the hip's ball-and-socket joint)
- the acetabulum (the indentation in the pelvis that forms the socket of the ball-and-socket joint)
- the greater trochanter (a protrusion on the upper part of the femur to which a number of muscles attach).

### Ligaments

The hip joint is surrounded by a strong joint capsule made up of four ligaments, the most important of which is the iliofemoral ligament. These tissues keep you from moving the hip to an extreme position that could dislocate the joint (pull the ball out of the socket).

### Cartilage

The hips have two kinds of cartilage:
- Articular cartilage coats the bones within the joint itself—specifically, the femoral head and the acetabulum (the ball and socket).
- The socket is further cushioned and deepened by a vital rim of cartilage called the labrum. The labrum helps keep the joint fixed in place and lubricated.

Additional lubrication in the joint comes in the form of synovial fluid from the lining of the joint capsule (the synovium). Thanks to the perfect fit of the bones in the joint, along with the slick articular

## Figure 2: Hip anatomy

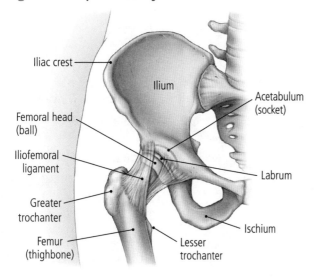

- Iliac crest
- Ilium
- Acetabulum (socket)
- Femoral head (ball)
- Iliofemoral ligament
- Labrum
- Greater trochanter
- Ischium
- Femur (thighbone)
- Lesser trochanter

The hip joint forms where the head of the femur fits into the acetabulum, or socket of the pelvis. A rim made of rubbery cartilage, called the labrum, surrounds the hip joint and keeps it lubricated. Muscles attach to the hip at a bony knob called the greater trochanter. Others attach at the lesser trochanter, just below it.

cartilage and the synovial fluid lubricating the space between them, the friction between the ball and socket in a healthy hip is less than that of two ice cubes rubbing together.

### Muscles

Muscles in the thigh and lower back help stabilize the hip and move the upper leg at the hip joint (see Figure 6, page 16).

- The quadriceps muscles in the front of the thigh help you lift your leg—for example, when you climb stairs.
- The hamstrings in the back of the leg extend the hip—for example, helping you straighten your leg again when climbing stairs.
- The iliopsoas (a muscle complex that runs from the lower back to the front of the thigh) helps flex the hip when you lift your leg to the front. It is one of several muscles known as hip flexors, which also include the rectus femoris, sartorius, and pectineus.
- The abductor muscles (gluteus medius, gluteus minimus, piriformis, and tensor fasciae latae) in the thigh move your legs out away from your body, so you can pull your leg out of bed or swing it over a motorcycle to climb aboard.
- Adductors (including the adductors longus, brevis, and magnus) pull your leg in toward your body.
- The large gluteus maximus muscle in the buttock extends the hip when you move your leg backward or to the side.

### Bursae

Places in the hip where tendons, muscles, and bones meet are protected by small, liquid-filled sacs called bursae. The body has more than 150 of these cushioning sacs, which reduce friction between bones and soft tissues. In the hip, there are three (see Figure 3, page 9).

## Bursitis

Although the bursae (see above) are designed to reduce friction around joints, they can become irritated, leading to a problem known as bursitis. The suffix *–itis* means inflammation. Thus, bursitis is inflammation of a bursa.

Often it is the bursa covering the greater trochanter that is affected, resulting in greater trochanteric pain syndrome (also known as trochanteric bursitis; see Figure 3, page 9). Greater trochanteric pain syndrome can result from a hard fall on your hip or the accumulation of minor stresses—such as small inju-

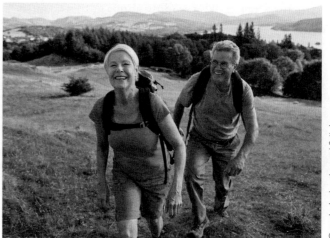

Climbing is no simple task. It requires mutiple sets of muscles—the quadriceps, hamstrings, hip flexors, and gluteal muscles—to work together, alternately contracting and relaxing in coordination.

ries, excess pressure on one hip when you walk (from scoliosis, other joint damage, or unequal leg lengths), or even from lying on one side for an extended period, such as after another injury that requires bed rest. Or, like other forms of bursitis, it may develop for no apparent reason.

Less often, people develop ischial bursitis, which occurs when the bursa under one of the ischia (the bones you sit on) becomes inflamed. As suggested by its nicknames "weaver's bottom" and "tailor's seat," it can occur from prolonged sitting on a hard surface, as well as from a fall or repeated friction during bicycling or rowing.

The iliopsoas bursa—the protective sac that lies between the front of the hip joint and the iliopsoas muscle, one of the hip flexors—can also be affected. Iliopsoas bursitis can be associated with rheumatoid arthritis or osteoarthritis of the hip, or with overdoing activities that require repeated hip flexing (such as soccer, ballet, jumping hurdles, or running uphill).

## Diagnosing hip bursitis

Your doctor will examine your hip, feeling for tender areas. In some cases, you may need an imaging test such as an x-ray or magnetic resonance imaging (MRI) to rule out a fracture, arthritis, or another painful hip condition.

## Treating hip bursitis

Treatment for hip bursitis starts by avoiding whatever activity triggered the pain and inflammation. You can help control the pain by taking an over-the-counter anti-inflammatory pain reliever—such as aspirin, ibuprofen (Advil, Motrin), or naproxen (Aleve)—or applying cold or heat to the inflamed hip. Your doc-

## ▶ Symptoms of hip bursitis

**For greater trochanteric pain syndrome:**
- Aching or burning on the outside of the upper thigh
- Pain that moves down the outside of the thigh to the knee
- Increasing pain when you push on or lie on the affected side
- Pain that interferes with sleep
- Pain triggered by walking, climbing stairs, or getting up from sitting

**For ischial bursitis:**
- Dull or sharp pain in the lower buttock
- Pain that increases when you sit down (especially on a hard surface) or lie on your back

**For iliopsoas bursitis:**
- Pain in the front of the hip that worsens when you flex the hip
- Radiating pain down the front of your thigh
- Limping (if only one leg is involved) or taking smaller steps
- Limited range of motion in the hip

## Figure 3: Bursitis

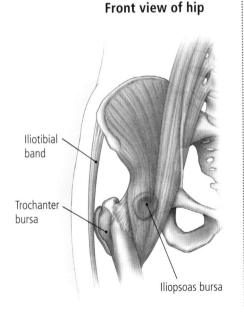
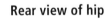
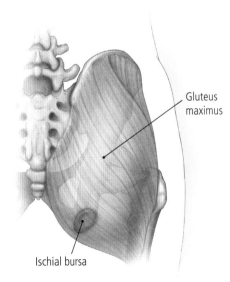

**Front view of hip**

**Rear view of hip**

Iliotibial band

Trochanter bursa

Iliopsoas bursa

Gluteus maximus

Ischial bursa

The hip has several fluid-filled sacs, called bursae, that cushion the joint. When one of these sacs becomes irritated or inflamed, the condition is known as bursitis. Inflammation of the trochanter bursa at the widest part of the hip is the most common type of bursitis in the hip. But inflammation can also occur at the iliopsoas bursa near the groin and the ischial bursa that you sit on.

tor may send you to a physical therapist to teach you exercises that strengthen your hip muscles as well as stretches to relieve tension in the hip.

For longer-term pain relief, you can see your doctor for a corticosteroid injection directly into the trochanter bursa. (Injection into an iliopsoas or ischial bursa requires imaging to guide the needle placement, which may require you to see a specialist.) These injections can continue to relieve pain for a few months.

After treatment, be careful to avoid or modify whatever activity caused the bursitis so you don't develop it again in the future.

Rarely is surgery necessary unless the bursitis results from an infection (which is rare).

# Groin pull (strain)

The area that we call the groin sits at the junction between the abdomen and thigh. A groin pull, or strain, typically involves stretching or tearing the adductor muscles, on the inside of the hip and thigh. These muscles help stabilize the trunk and pull the legs inward. Groin injuries are common in people who play sports that involve running, jumping, and quick movements or direction changes, such as soccer, football, skiing, track and field, and hockey. You might suffer a groin strain while sprinting off the starting block in a track race, or shooting a goal in hockey (in

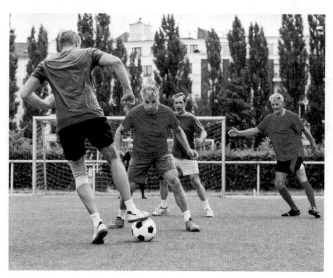

It's not unusual for people who play sports involving running, jumping, and quick changes of direction to pull their groin muscles (the adductor muscles on the inside of the hip and thigh).

fact, groin strains make up 10% of all hockey injuries). However, you don't need to be an athlete to strain your groin. Lifting something heavy or slipping while you walk can also cause this injury.

## Diagnosing a groin pull

Your doctor will apply slight pressure to the affected leg to check for pain, and will also look for bruising and other symptoms that indicate a groin pull. An MRI can help confirm the diagnosis and rule out conditions with similar symptoms; however, this imaging test is usually unnecessary to diagnose a groin pull.

Doctors assign one of the following three grades to groin strains based on the degree of muscle damage that occurs:

- **Grade 1** is a partial stretch, or a tear of a few muscle fibers. You'll have some tenderness, but you should still be able to walk and use the affected leg.
- **Grade 2** is a moderate stretch or tear of a larger number of muscle fibers. You'll have pain, loss of strength, and trouble walking.
- **Grade 3** is a severe tear. Sometimes the muscle rips completely. You'll see bruising under the skin in the area of the tear. It will be very painful and difficult for you to use the affected leg.

## Treating a groin pull

You'll need to rest the affected leg to give it time to heal. Apply a cold pack to the injured area for 15 or 20 minutes at a time, up to every two hours for the first couple of days. (Note: you should never apply ice directly to the skin; instead, place a thin towel between

> ## Symptoms of a groin pull
>
> - A popping feeling or noise when the injury occurs
> - Sharp or throbbing pain in the groin and the inside of the thigh
> - Pain that intensifies when you raise your knee, pull your legs together, or move your legs apart
> - Muscle spasms in the groin
> - Bruising in the thigh or groin area
> - Weakness in the leg when you try to walk or climb stairs
> - Limping when you walk

© alvarez | Getty Images

them to avoid skin damage.) An over-the-counter anti-inflammatory pain reliever—such as aspirin, ibuprofen, or naproxen—can help keep you comfortable while the injury heals. As soon as you have healed enough, your doctor may refer you to a physical therapist. The therapist will work you through a number of exercises to strengthen the muscles around your hip and prevent another groin injury in the future.

# Hip fracture

For thousands of people who break a hip, life is never the same again. As many as half will no longer be able to walk without assistance—even if they were healthy and mobile beforehand. One in five people over age 50 dies within a year of a hip fracture from ensuing health complications.

The two most common types of hip fracture involve the thighbone (femur):

- **A femoral neck fracture** occurs in the horizontal section of the thighbone, about one to two inches from the ball of the hip joint (see Figure 2, page 8).
- **An intertrochanteric fracture** occurs in the thighbone three to four inches below the ball of the hip.

Fractures of the hip socket, which are considered to be pelvic fractures, are less common.

### Diagnosing a hip fracture

A possible hip fracture needs immediate evaluation. As x-ray is likely to show a fracture if one exists. But if it doesn't and your symptoms strongly suggest a fracture, MRI may reveal a break that has not moved out of place or a fracture involving the hip socket.

### Treating a hip fracture

The goal of treatment is to reconnect the broken bone and hold it in place, so the hip works properly until it can heal—about three months. Surgery within 24 hours is usually necessary to make this repair. If you must wait for the operation, the hip may be held in traction (using weights to extend the muscles around the hip) while you wait.

If you have a femoral neck fracture in which the pieces are not displaced, the orthopedic surgeon may connect the bone with surgical screws. If the bone has

▶ **Symptoms of a hip fracture**
- Severe pain in the hip or groin
- A deformed appearance to the hip, or a turned-out leg that may appear shorter than the other
- Swelling, tenderness and bruising around the hip
- Inability to stand up, or a hip too weak to lift the leg

moved well out of place, or if you are older and not active, he or she may replace the head of the femur with a metal device, a procedure called a partial hip replacement. Or, if arthritis is present, the surgeon may perform a total hip replacement (see Figure 5, page 13).

After surgery, it can take several months for the hip to heal completely. The goal of rehabilitation is to get you back on your feet as soon as possible.

# Osteoarthritis

The word arthritis comes from *arthron*, the Greek word for "joint," and *–itis*, a suffix denoting inflammation. There are more than 100 types of arthritis, but osteoarthritis—the so-called wear-and-tear form of

---

## Figure 4: Osteoarthritic changes in the hip

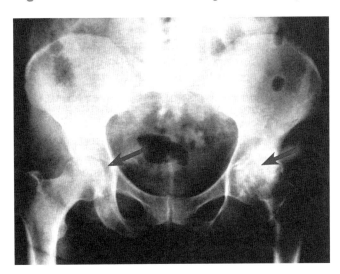

This x-ray shows what happens when osteoarthritis affects the hip—in this case, the patient's left hip (shown on the right side of the image). Compared with the visible outline of the ball-and-socket joint on the opposite side, the joint on this side has noticeably deteriorated.

arthritis—is the best known. It is also the most common form of degenerative joint disease, affecting more than 30 million adults in the United States. Weight-bearing joints like the hips and knees are most commonly affected. One or both hips may have arthritis.

Osteoarthritis begins with degeneration of the articular cartilage that normally helps cushion the joint. As the protective cartilage is worn away, the space between the femur ball and the hip socket narrows (see Figure 4, page 11). As a result, the bones of the hip joint rub painfully against one another. New bone begins to grow as a reaction to the joint degeneration, forming bone spurs (known medically as osteophytes).

## Finding the assistive device that fits you

After an injury to your hip or leg, or if you have a mobility-compromising condition like arthritis, an assistive device such as a cane or walker can be invaluable for helping you get around and keeping you safely active. These devices take some of the weight off the painful leg, increase stability, and improve your balance.

It's important when you do select a cane or another mobility aid that you get the right fit. One study found that more than two-thirds of people with canes have ones that are damaged, the wrong height, or otherwise inappropriate for them. For example, a long cane will put too much pressure on your arms, while a short one will force you to lean forward in an unnatural position. For help in getting fitted for one of these devices, see your doctor.

**Standard canes** typically come in wood or aluminum, with a curved or *T*-shaped handle. They're reasonably priced and lightweight. Some fold for easier storage. A standard cane will improve your base of support, but it won't bear a lot of weight. This type of cane can be helpful if you have arthritis in only one hip or one knee, and you haven't lost your ability to balance.

**Offset canes** have a handle that curves away from and then toward you to distribute your weight over the cane. They're designed to support more weight than a standard cane, and they may be helpful if you have painful arthritis in your hip or knee.

**Multiple-leg canes** have three or four legs. They provide more support and can bear more weight than a standard or offset cane, and may be useful to people who have difficulty balancing. Plus, they're freestanding, in case you need to use one or both of your hands. Because all legs of the cane need to be firmly on the ground for stability, you may walk more slowly with this type of cane.

**Standard walkers** have four rubber-tipped legs. This is the most stable type of walker, but also the slowest, because you'll need to pick it up and put it down as you walk. Walkers are ideal for people with arthritis of the knees and hips on both sides of the body, weakness in both legs, and more significant balance issues. Yet you'll need the upper-body strength to pick up and put down the walker with each step.

**Two-wheeled walkers** have two wheels in the front and two rubber-tipped legs in the back. They provide easier movement than a standard walker, while still offering a good amount of stability.

**Four-wheeled walkers (rollators)** most closely allow you to replicate your normal walk, and they may be preferable for people who have trouble lifting and setting down a standard walker. You can move more quickly with four wheels than you would with a standard walker, but a wheeled walker won't bear as much of your weight.

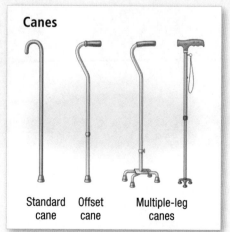

**Canes**

Standard cane    Offset cane    Multiple-leg canes

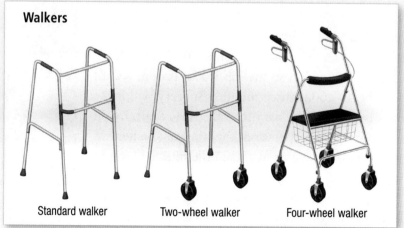

**Walkers**

Standard walker      Two-wheel walker      Four-wheel walker

Osteoarthritis tends to appear later in life. As you get into your 60s and beyond, osteoarthritis may cause joint aching and stiffness, especially when you first wake up in the morning or after you've been in the same position for a while (such as after a long drive). The discomfort will likely increase until you take steps to manage your arthritis.

While osteoarthritis has long been considered an age-related disease, we now know that genes, obesity, injury, inflammation, and other factors may contribute to its development. You can't stop the aging process or change your genes, but you do have control over your weight, which is the leading modifiable risk factor for osteoarthritis. The hips are weight-bearing joints, and the more weight they have to bear, the more stress the bones and cartilage will endure. People who are obese are nearly seven times more likely to develop osteoarthritis than those who are at a normal weight. The extra weight strains joints and makes it harder to exercise. A lack of exercise deconditions joints further and leads to even more weight gain. And the painful cycle continues.

## Diagnosing hip osteoarthritis

Your primary care doctor can serve as your first point of contact if you suspect you have osteoarthritis. Later, you might also see a rheumatologist and possibly an orthopedic specialist. During the exam, your doctor will look for signs like pain, limited range of

### ▶ Symptoms of hip osteoarthritis

- Pain in your thigh or groin that may radiate to your buttocks
- Stiffness in the hip
- Reduced range of motion in the hip
- A grinding or popping feeling when you move the joint

motion in the hip joint, and problems with your gait (the way you walk). An x-ray can reveal narrowing of the joint space, bone spurs, and damage to the cartilage that are the hallmark signs of osteoarthritis (see Figure 4, page 11).

## Treating hip osteoarthritis

Your doctor will typically start you on the most conservative measures first. The goal is to relieve your pain without causing unnecessary side effects. Exercise is one strategy that offers pain relief with little risk. A combination of low-impact aerobic activities like walking and bike riding, as well as resistance training, helps with weight loss and may strengthen the muscles that support your hip joint and improve range of motion. A physical therapist can help design a program that's well-suited to your needs and abilities. Water exercise is among the best choices for arthritis because the buoyancy of water takes pressure off sore joints. A local chapter of the Arthritis Foundation may offer classes in your area (see "Resources," page 52).

Medication is another option. Acetaminophen (Tylenol) or an over-the-counter nonsteroidal anti-inflammatory drug (NSAID) such as aspirin, ibuprofen, or naproxen may help. Prescription versions of many of these drugs are also available. But because NSAIDs can cause side effects such as stomach ulcers, gastrointestinal bleeding, heart attack, or stroke, do not use these drugs on a daily basis unless recommended and

## Figure 5: Total hip replacement surgery

When rough and damaged cartilage prevents the bones of the hip from moving smoothly, an orthopedic surgeon can install an artificial joint with two parts. The head of the thighbone (femur) is replaced with an artificial ball with a long stem that fits down inside the bone. This part of the prosthesis is called the femoral component. The other part of the prosthesis, called the acetabular cup, fits inside the hip socket. Cement may be applied, depending on which type of artificial joint is used. The two pieces fit smoothly together to restore comfortable ball-in-socket movement.

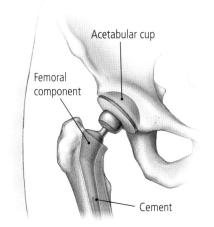

Acetabular cup

Femoral component

Cement

monitored by your doctor. Acetaminophen, too, may cause problems. It can cause liver damage if you regularly exceed the maximum dose of 3,000 milligrams. Using a combination of acetaminophen and an NSAID can help you take a lower dose of each pain reliever.

For a more powerful anti-inflammatory effect, your doctor may inject a corticosteroid medication directly into the affected joint. This approach is used only when absolutely necessary—and usually no more than two or three times a year—because frequent injections of these drugs can damage a joint and may increase the risk of infection.

Taking pressure off the joint can also help. If hip arthritis makes it hard for you to get around, a cane, walker, or other assistive device could be key to maintaining your independence and preventing a fall. Hold a cane in the hand opposite your bad hip. (For tips on selecting a device that suits your needs, see "Finding the assistive device that fits you," page 12.)

Surgery is always a last resort, but it may become necessary if your hip pain doesn't improve with other treatments. Two procedures are available to fix the damage of hip osteoarthritis: hip resurfacing and total hip replacement. A total hip replacement removes the damaged femur head and socket and replaces them with prosthetic versions made from metal or ceramic (see Figure 5, page 13). In hip resurfacing, the surgeon removes damaged bone and cartilage from the hip socket and replaces it with a metal cup. The femur head is left intact, but it is covered in a layer of smooth metal.

Both procedures come with possible risks, including infection, excess bleeding, and blood clots. A resurfaced hip offers the advantages of being less likely to dislocate and providing a total return to activities like running and climbing, which may make it preferable for younger, more active people. Yet there are downsides to resurfacing, too. As the metal surfaces of ball and socket interact, they can potentially release harmful metal into the blood. A resurfaced hip is also more likely to fracture, especially in women whose bones are weakened from osteoporosis. For these reasons, resurfacing is typically reserved for younger men who have strong bones.

▶ **Symptoms of hip tendinitis**

- Pain in the front of your hip, especially when you bend your hip or raise your leg
- Soreness in the groin area when you touch it (because the iliopsoas tendon sits close to the skin)
- A snapping or clicking sensation when you walk

# Tendinitis

A tendon is a specialized part of a muscle that connects the muscle to a bone. Inflammation in the tendon that connects the iliopsoas muscle (the main hip flexor muscle) to the upper thigh is known as hip flexor tendinitis. (Damage from microscopic tears and degeneration is known as hip flexor tendinosis. The umbrella term covering both hip tendinitis and tendinosis is hip flexor tendinopathy, but most people just refer to both as tendinitis.)

Hip tendinitis often affects people who play sports that involve repetitive hip movements, particularly cyclists, runners, swimmers, triathletes, dancers, and tennis players. In older people, it tends to affect those whose gait has been thrown off by related problems in the spine, knees, ankles, or hips. An injury such as a fall can also injure the tendon in the hip.

## Diagnosing hip tendinitis

Your doctor will ask about your symptoms and whether you participate in any activities that might have contributed to tendinitis. Typically, the diagnosis can be made from symptoms alone, without the need for an MRI scan.

## Treating hip tendinitis

Rest the hip to give it a chance to heal. Avoid any sports or other activities that might have contributed to the injury. To reduce pain and swelling, hold an ice pack to your hip for 15 or 20 minutes at a time, a few times a day. An over-the-counter anti-inflammatory pain reliever such as aspirin, ibuprofen, or naproxen can also be helpful for pain and swelling. Corticosteroid injections can provide more sustained pain relief. Once the immediate injury has healed, work with a physical therapist to regain the strength in your hip muscles. ♥

# Upper leg pain

Your upper legs are where you'll find some of the strongest muscles in your body. These muscles power your movements, whether you're climbing the stairs, getting up from a chair, or jumping hurdles on a track. But as strong as they are, these muscles can suffer injury. You can strain, tear, or otherwise damage the muscles themselves or their tendons as the result of overuse, repetitive motions, accidents, sudden movements that wrench your leg, or exercising without properly warming up first.

The nerves that supply feeling to the upper leg or that run through it can also cause unpleasant sensations in the upper leg, ranging from pain to numbness and tingling. And redness or swelling in the thigh after surgery or a long period of immobility could indicate a blockage in one of the leg's deep veins.

This chapter reviews some of the leading causes of upper leg pain (listed in alphabetical order), along with the methods used to diagnose and treat them. The chapter begins with a review of upper leg anatomy.

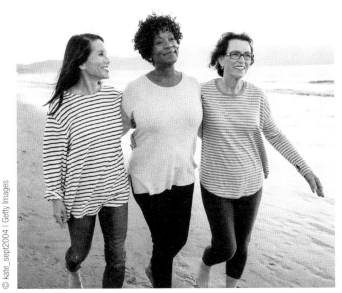

The powerful quadriceps muscles in the front of your thighs work just about every time you use your legs. The hamstring muscles in the back of your thighs help control their movements.

## Upper leg anatomy 101

When it comes to providing the raw power for locomotion, the upper legs play the starring role. It takes all their anatomical structures working in tandem to make that happen. Following is a quick rundown.

### Bone

No complicated anatomy lesson is necessary here. There is one bone in the upper leg—the thighbone (femur). As noted earlier, it is both the longest and strongest bone in the body. It takes significant force to break the shaft of the femur, helping to explain why motor vehicle accidents are the leading cause of femur fractures. The upper end of the thighbone fits into the hip socket. The lower end forms the upper portion of the knee joint.

### Muscles

The musculature of the upper leg is more complicated than the bone structure. It includes several important muscle groups.

**Quadriceps.** Covering the front of the thigh is a large group of muscles known as the quadriceps (see Figure 6, page 16). *Quad-* comes from the Latin word for "four." The name is well suited, given that this muscle group has four parts: the rectus femoris, vastus lateralis, vastus medialis, and vastus intermedius. The quadriceps starts at the hip bone and attaches to the kneecap. Its muscles work just about every time you use your legs, whether you're straightening your knees, standing up, or walking.

**Hamstrings.** Running down the back of each thigh from the bottom of the pelvis to just below the knee are the three hamstring muscles: the semitendinosus, semimembranosus, and biceps femoris. They are responsible for movements of the hip and knee, allowing you to bend your knee and extend your leg.

**Iliopsoas.** The iliopsoas muscle is a powerful, hardworking muscle that flexes the hip joint and lifts the knee whenever you walk or run. The strongest of the four muscles known as hip flexors, the iliopsoas is formed from the junction of two muscles—the psoas major and iliacus—which begin at the lower spine, cross the hip joint, and then connect into one band in the thigh. A tendon attaches this merged muscle to the thighbone at the lesser trochanter, a small bony projection below the greater trochanter (see Figure 2, page 8). A tight iliopsoas muscle sometimes causes pain in the lower back, a deception that has earned this muscle the nickname "hidden prankster."

**Adductors and abductors.** The word adductor derives from the Latin prefix *ad-*, for "toward," and *ducere*, which means "to lead." The word perfectly captures movement of the adductor muscles—pulling one leg in toward the other. Their opposing muscles, the abductors, pull the legs away from each other and rotate them outward. If you've ever used abductor and adductor machines at the gym, you've seen these two muscle groups at work.

**Gluteal muscles.** Bringing up the rear (literally), are the three gluteal muscles that make up the buttocks: gluteus maximus, gluteus medius, and gluteus minimus. The gluteus maximus is by far the largest of these three muscles. Together, this muscle trio helps to control movement in the hip and thigh. You'll use them whenever you climb stairs, stand up from a squatting position, or run.

## Nerves

Running down from the lower back through the buttocks and down the back of each leg to the feet is the sciatic nerve. It's the longest nerve in the body and supplies feeling to the legs. Pressure on this nerve from a herniated disc, narrowed spine, or other medical condition creates the numbness, tin-gling, and pain known as sciatica (see page 23).

Other nerves in the upper leg include the following:

**Common peroneal nerve.** This branch of the sciatic nerve provides feeling to the front and sides of the legs and activates the muscles that flex the toes.

**Femoral nerve.** It provides feeling to the front of the thigh and activates the muscles that allow the knee to extend.

**Lateral femoral cutaneous nerve.** This nerve is part of the lumbar plexus, a network of nerves in the lower back. It provides feeling to the front and sides of the thighs.

## Blood vessels

A network of arteries delivers blood to the legs. Chief among them is the femoral artery, the main artery in the thigh. Because this artery is large and easy to feel through the skin, hospital clinicians often use it as an insertion point for catheters that can be snaked through the arteries to other parts of the body, to help diagnose and sometimes treat problems involving the

## Figure 6: Anatomy of the thighs

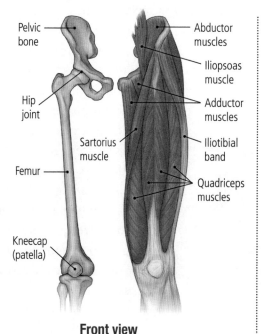
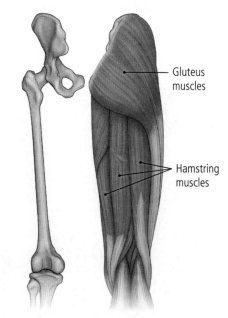

Pelvic bone

Abductor muscles

Iliopsoas muscle

Hip joint

Adductor muscles

Sartorius muscle

Iliotibial band

Femur

Quadriceps muscles

Gluteus muscles

Hamstring muscles

Kneecap (patella)

**Front view**

**Rear view**

The quadriceps are usually treated as a single unit, but there are actually four quadriceps muscles at the front of the thigh. In the back of the thigh, there are three hamstrings. In addition, a variety of muscles known as hip flexors, abductors, and adductors help you to move your leg as you want to.

heart, brain, and kidneys. Although the femoral artery can suffer from peripheral artery disease (PAD; see "Peripheral artery disease and claudication," page 43), PAD more often affects smaller arteries in the lower legs.

Veins return blood to the heart. They can be either deep inside muscles (deep veins) or near the surface of the skin (superficial veins). Deep veins carry more blood and can potentially be involved in more serious problems than superficial veins (see "Deep-vein thrombosis," below). Much of the blood from superficial veins eventually flows into the deep veins.

## Deep-vein thrombosis (DVT)

Deep veins are the major blood vessels that carry 90% or more of blood away from the legs and back to the heart. As discussed earlier (see "Leg anatomy: An overview," page 2), tiny one-way valves in the leg veins close as blood passes through, in order to propel blood upward against gravity, thereby preventing it from flowing backward. But muscles surrounding the deep veins also assist by squeezing the veins—a pumping action that helps propel blood upward toward the heart. Prolonged inactivity—for example, sitting in a cramped position for an extended time—can cause blood flow in the deep veins to become sluggish, which in turn encourages blood to coagulate, forming a blood clot (thrombus). The condition is known as deep-vein thrombosis, or DVT.

DVT causes pain, redness, and swelling in the leg, as blood flow is blocked by the clot, and blood pools behind it. But complications of DVT can be far worse than that. DVT can have stealthy and sometimes deadly consequences, when a blood clot that forms in the leg travels up to the lungs and becomes lodged in an artery there, preventing blood from reaching the lungs. Pulmonary embolism, as this problem is known, is a serious complication of DVT. These two conditions are known collectively as venous thromboembolism, or VTE.

Another problem associated with DVT is the damage that the buildup of blood behind the clot can do to the little valves in the leg veins. This damage leads to a complication called post-thrombotic syn-

> ## Symptoms of deep-vein thrombosis (DVT)
>
> A clot in a deep vein causes these symptoms:
>
> • pain in the upper leg or calf
> • red, swollen skin on the leg
> • warmth over the leg.
>
> If the condition progresses to pulmonary embolism, you may have the following symptoms:
>
> • shortness of breath
> • chest pain that may get worse when you inhale or cough
> • lightheadedness, dizziness, feeling as though you're about to pass out
> • rapid heart rate
> • coughing up blood.
>
> Pulmonary embolism can be life-threatening. If you have these symptoms, ask for medical assistance, call 911, or go to an emergency room right away.

drome, which is characterized by pain, swelling, color changes, and sometimes open sores. About 40% of people who suffer DVT will develop some degree of post-thrombotic syndrome, and in about 8% the condition will become severe enough to be disabling.

DVT is perhaps best known for developing during long airplane flights, giving rise to the nickname "economy class syndrome." But a recent study of Japanese people fleeing a 2016 earthquake also documented an "epidemic" of leg clots among earthquake victims who couldn't find room in shelters and had to spend the night in their cars. Extended immobility for other reasons—such as prolonged bed rest following surgery or an injury—can also lead to DVT.

Other potential causes or risk factors for clotting in the deep veins of the upper leg include

• older age (over 65)
• diseases such as cancer, heart disease, heart failure, lung disease, and inflammatory bowel disease (Crohn's disease and ulcerative colitis)
• inherited blood clotting disorders (inherited thrombophilia)
• direct damage to leg veins (for example, from injury or surgery)

- obesity (which leads to higher pressure on large veins, changes in blood chemistry, and other changes)
- smoking (which leads to changes in the lining of blood vessels)
- the use of birth control pills or hormone therapy (which can affect clotting)
- pregnancy (the risk continues for three months after giving birth).

As many as 900,000 Americans experience DVT in any given year, and up to one in nine die from it.

## Diagnosing DVT

If you have symptoms of DVT, get to a hospital emergency room as soon as possible. If your doctor thinks you have DVT after performing an exam and getting a rundown of your symptoms, he or she may recommend a D-dimer blood test and ultrasound or another imaging test right away to conclusively diagnose it. D-dimer is a protein that tends to increase when your body forms blood clots. However, it's not a perfect test: other conditions may cause an elevation in this test, and not everyone with a DVT has an elevated level of D-dimer.

Lower-extremity ultrasound is a test that uses sound waves to visualize the flow of blood and detect clots in your leg veins. A technician runs a transducer over your leg; this device releases sound waves, which bounce off of structures inside your leg to create an image on a monitor.

## Treating DVT

Anticoagulants, or blood thinners, are the main treatment for DVT. They don't dissolve the clot, but they prevent new clots from forming and the initial clot from growing larger while the body breaks it down. Initial anticoagulation treatment usually includes an injected medication (such as heparin or fondaparinux) or an oral drug such as rivaroxaban (Xarelto) or apixaban (Eliquis), followed by another three months of oral medication, such as warfarin (Coumadin). The cause of your DVT will determine the length of your treatment. If the DVT developed because of bed rest after surgery or another known and reversible risk, you may only need to stay on these medications for three months. But if the cause is unknown and you may have a chronic clotting problem, treatment could take six to 12 months, or even continue indefinitely.

Once you've had an episode of DVT, your risk of another one increases. About 30% of people who've had either DVT or a pulmonary embolism will have a second one within 10 years (see "How to prevent DVT," at left).

---

### How to prevent DVT

To avoid DVT, observe the following precautions:

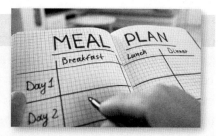

- On long flights, get up and walk around every two to three hours. While you sit, exercise your legs by alternately squeezing and releasing your leg muscles, circling your feet, and pointing and flexing your toes.

- On long car trips, stop every couple of hours to stretch and walk around.

- After surgery, get up and move as soon as you are allowed to. Some hospitals use intermittent pneumatic compression devices to prevent blood clots from forming after surgical procedures. These devices look like large cuffs or leg warmers that alternately fill with air and squeeze your legs to keep blood circulating.

- During pregnancy, stay active. Try to walk every day, and avoid prolonged bed rest. Stay hydrated. Drinking plenty of water can help keep your blood from thickening to the point where it forms clots.

- If you smoke, ask your doctor about nicotine replacement products, medication, therapy, and other methods to help you quit.

- If you're overweight, get help to lose the weight from a dietitian or a structured program like Weight Watchers or Jenny Craig.

You can also ask your doctor about compression stockings. These hose-like stockings exert constant pressure on the legs to keep blood flowing. The research on compression stockings in people who have had DVT has been mixed—some studies suggest it prevents post-thrombotic syndrome, while others have not found a benefit. Some people find these stockings uncomfortable and unattractive. If your doctor suggests that you wear them, you may reduce the discomfort by having them custom-fit, so that they're not too tight, too long, too hot, or the like.

# Hamstring strain or tear

Located at the back of the leg, the hamstring muscles run down the back of each thigh and across two joints—the hip and knee—enabling you to bend your knee and straighten your leg at the hip. Together with the quadriceps at the front of the thigh and the gluteal muscles in your buttocks, the hamstrings alternately contract and relax so that you can walk, climb stairs, get up out of a chair, and perform a host of other actions. They also provide the speed and agility you need to be competitive on the sporting field.

However, quick movements and sudden stops while playing sports such as tennis, basketball, track, or soccer can stretch these bands of tissue to the point of injury—either overstretching (a strain, or pull) or an actual rip in the muscle (a hamstring tear). The hamstrings are more vulnerable to injury than the quadriceps, in part because of imbalances in strength between the two muscle groups. The quadriceps are usually stronger, so the hamstrings may fatigue faster, setting up the possibility of strains. Overworked, fatigued hamstrings are also more vulnerable to tearing, because they can't absorb as much energy during exertion. Muscle overload is another hazard, which occurs when you suddenly put the full weight of your body onto the muscle as it is lengthening—for example, as you push off a starting block into a sprint.

In fact, the hamstrings are among the most commonly injured muscles in athletes. Hamstring injuries account for 37% of all muscle injuries in professional soccer players, and they are responsible for 25% of missed games among athletes over all. That said, anyone can suffer a hamstring injury when placing large, sudden demands on these muscles—for example, when dashing for the bus. These injuries often happen when people have not warmed up before a workout or when their quads are much stronger than their hamstrings, setting up an imbalance in how the two muscle groups work with each other.

Most hamstring injuries affect the thick center portion of the muscle.

## Diagnosing a hamstring strain or tear

During the exam, your doctor will gently press on the back of your thigh, looking for tenderness and swell-

▶ **Symptoms of a severe hamstring strain or tear**

- Sudden, sharp pain in the back of the thigh
- A popping sensation
- Swelling in the first few hours after the injury
- Bruises on the back of your upper leg
- Weakness and difficulty bearing weight on the injured leg

ing. The doctor may ask you to move your leg into specific positions to determine exactly which muscle you've injured.

Hamstring strains range in severity from a mild strain to a complete tear:

- **Grade 1** is the least severe type of strain, in which the muscle is overstretched.
- **Grade 2** is a partial tear.
- **Grade 3** is a complete tear of the muscle from its connection to bone. In the worst-case scenario, the torn hamstring pulls part of the bone away with it (an avulsion fracture). An x-ray, ultrasound, or MRI can identify muscle tears and avulsion fractures; however, these tests are not usually necessary.

## Treating a hamstring strain or tear

Treatment for a hamstring muscle strain or tear follows the same general protocol as for many other sports-related injuries: rest, ice, compression, elevation (RICE).

- **Rest.** Avoid the activity that caused the injury. Depending on the extent of the pull, your doctor might recommend that you use crutches to take weight off the affected leg until it heals.
- **Ice.** Hold an ice pack to the hamstring for about 20 minutes at a time, several times a day. Wrap the ice in a towel to avoid injuring your skin.
- **Compression.** Wrap the leg in a bandage to keep down the swelling.
- **Elevation.** Prop up your leg on a pillow. Raising the leg helps move fluid back toward your heart, which brings down swelling.

An over-the-counter anti-inflammatory drug such as aspirin, ibuprofen (Advil, Motrin), or naproxen (Aleve) may be useful for easing pain right after the injury, although research hasn't shown that these pain relievers help with healing.

Once the muscle has healed, your doctor might refer you for physical therapy. There, you'll learn exercises to improve your mobility, increase your range of motion, and rebuild strength in your upper leg muscles. Your doctor and physical therapist will let you know when it's safe to return to sports and other physical activities.

If you have a total muscle or tendon tear—or an avulsion fracture, in which a tendon rips away from the bone, bringing a piece of the bone with it—you may need surgery to fix it. During this procedure, the surgeon pulls the hamstring muscle back into place and secures it to the bone with stitches or sutures. A tear in the muscle is stitched together. Because of the severity of the injury, it can take about six months to rehabilitate and recover.

A relatively new treatment called platelet-rich plasma (PRP) injection is currently under investigation for treating hamstring injuries. Along with red and white blood cells, platelets are a component of the liquid portion of blood (plasma). Platelets not only help your blood clot, but they also promote healing after an injury. To prepare the PRP, a small amount of your blood is removed from a vein. It is then spun in a centrifuge to separate out the platelets. Plasma enriched with platelets is then injected back into the muscle. Early evidence suggests this treatment could speed healing, although the research isn't conclusive at this point. The treatment also isn't usually covered by insurance.

Unfortunately, hamstring injuries are often not a one-time occurrence. One out of every three people who suffers one of these injuries will have another one, sometimes within the first two weeks after they return to the sport that caused it. To avoid future injuries, make sure you warm up before working out or playing sports—for example, by marching in place for several minutes first. After your workout, be sure to stretch your hamstrings. One way to do that is to sit on the floor with both legs extended in front of you. Slide your hands down your legs until you feel a slight pull in the backs of your legs. Hold for 30 seconds, and then return to an upright position.

▶ **Symptoms of iliotibial band syndrome**

- Pain along the iliotibial (IT) band, from the hip to below the knee
- Pain, swelling, warmth, or redness in the outer part of the knee
- Pain on the outside of the hip that is worsened by pressure, such as when lying on the affected side
- Pain when you start to exercise, but that improves as you warm up (eventually you may have pain even while at rest)
- Pain that gets worse when you run down hills or stairs, lengthen your stride, or sit for long periods of time with your knees bent

## Iliotibial band syndrome

The iliotibial (IT) band is a thick band of connective tissue that runs down the side of your upper leg, from the iliac crest of your hip bone to the outside of your knee. Alongside the knee, this band passes over the epicondyle, a bony bump at the outside of the lower end of your thighbone. A bursa keeps the movement of the IT band smooth over this bony protrusion and prevents friction as you walk or run. But when you repeatedly flex and extend your knee—for example, from running up and down hills or cycling for long periods of time—the IT band rubs back and forth against the epicondyle and gets irritated and swollen. Both the tendon and bursa can become inflamed and sore, a condition known as iliotibial band syndrome. The pain and tenderness may be confined to the outer part of your knee, or it can spread to the thigh and hip. A tight IT band can also cause people with hip problems to lose range of motion in the joint.

IT band syndrome affects up to 14% of runners. But the condition can occur in anyone who overdoes it while running, cycling, skiing, or playing soccer. You're more likely to develop IT band syndrome if you

- train intensively or for long periods of time (although this condition can also occur in people who exercise or play sports at more typical intensities and durations)
- don't warm up properly before an activity
- suddenly increase the intensity or frequency of your training sessions

- are in poor physical condition and suddenly start or return to physical activities
- use poor form when you run or play sports
- have a tighter-than-usual IT band
- have bowed legs (a space between your lower legs and knees when your feet are pressed together)
- have weak muscles in your knee or hip.

IT band syndrome is often a secondary problem, which means that it develops because of another injury or condition. Lower back or hip pain, for example, can cause a limp that leads to IT band syndrome, particularly in elderly people. The syndrome is more common in those who have tight IT bands, unbalanced leg muscle strength, high or low arches, or unequal leg lengths.

## Diagnosing iliotibial band syndrome

During the examination, your doctor will press on the outside of the leg or injured knee, looking for any tenderness and swelling. The doctor might move your knee into different positions to see if the IT band is tight. X-rays or other imaging tests aren't usually needed, but they may help your doctor rule out other conditions as possible causes of your pain.

## Treating iliotibial band syndrome

Most people can completely relieve IT band syndrome within six weeks by resting the knee. If you don't

give the injury enough time to heal, it can continue for much longer, and you may end up with chronic inflammation of your tendon and bursa. To relieve pain and inflammation, hold ice to your knee for 15 to 20 minutes at a time, once every two or three hours. Take over-the-counter anti-inflammatory pain relievers if you need them and your doctor says they're safe for you. Steroid injections are another option to relieve pain from IT band syndrome.

Your doctor will likely prescribe a physical therapy program that includes stretching and strengthening exercises to improve your balance, coordination, and posture (referred to collectively as neuromuscular re-education). In addition to working your knees and hips, the therapist will give you exercises to strengthen your core muscles—not just in your abdomen, but in your back and buttocks. Weakness in your core destabilizes your body and can contribute to IT band syndrome. Some therapists use manual therapy, in which they move certain muscles and joints that you may not be able to work yourself. Manual therapy helps to improve strength and range of motion.

Surgery is rarely necessary. The procedure to treat IT band syndrome removes part of the IT band, the bursa, or both. The IT band is then reattached to prevent it from rubbing against the bone on the side of your knee.

To prevent another episode of IT band syndrome in the future, make sure you warm up for at least five to 10 minutes before running, cycling, or doing other athletic activities. Try to avoid running up and down hills, or at least limit the time you spend on hills. And when you do run, wear good-quality shoes that properly support your feet (see "How to find the right running shoes," page 22). Also, stay on a consistent training schedule. If you have to stop training for several days or weeks, get back into your old routine gradually to avoid injury. And don't overtrain, but rather give yourself time to recover in between exercise sessions. Work with a trainer to learn the proper training techniques for your activity.

Finally, it's very important to stretch after exercising. That should include regular stretching of the IT band (see Figure 7, at left).

## Figure 7: Iliotibial band stretch

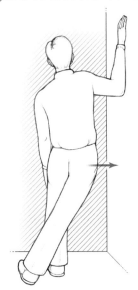

With your right arm against the wall for support, cross your right foot behind your left. With both feet on the floor, slowly lean your hip toward the wall. Hold for 20 seconds. Switch sides and repeat.

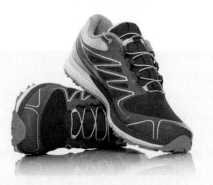

## How to find the right running shoes

Often, knee and leg problems result from overuse or an immediate injury. But sometimes, wearing the wrong running shoe contributes to poor body mechanics, which in turn leads to pain. Don't just choose whatever shoes are on sale. Have them fitted correctly, and make sure they're comfortable right away. Following are a few tips to help.

**Give your shoes an expiration date.** No matter how much you paid for them, running shoes won't last forever. With each step, you slowly wear out the material that cushions and protects your feet and legs. Plan to buy a new pair about once every 350 to 500 miles. For many people, that works out to a new pair about once every three to six months.

**Get fitted.** Many discount shoe stores make you find and fit your own running shoes. Take the time to go to a store where a knowledgeable salesperson will help you get the right fit. He or she can help you determine the best shoe for your foot shape and your style of running.

**Go for a test run.** Some stores have a treadmill you can use for a test run. Other stores without a treadmill might let you take the shoes outside for a run to help you decide. Make sure your heel doesn't slide up and down in the shoe while you run, and be sure your toes don't hit the front of the toe box. Give them some wiggle room.

**Decide what amount of cushioning you want.** If a traditional running shoe with a lot of cushioning is working well for you, then stick with it. The shoe should feel light in your hand but have enough flexibility to let your foot bend naturally.

**If you're getting repeated stress injuries, consider switching to a minimalist shoe.** These very light shoes, which have much thinner soles, are designed to shift your landing position from the heel to the middle or front of the foot, thereby lessening the heavy impact of a heel landing. If you do make the switch, dial back the number of miles you run at first and build back up gradually, in order to adjust to the new style of running and avoid new injuries.

**Consider special insoles.** If running is causing you pain, special shoe inserts made of gel, foam, or plastic can make a difference. These insoles are available at most stores that sell running shoes. Substitute them for the insole in the shoe.

# Meralgia paresthetica

Meralgia paresthetica is a condition marked by numbness, tingling, and burning in your outer thigh. "Meralgia" comes from the Greek words *meros*, meaning "thigh," and *algos*, meaning "pain." It's caused by pressure on the lateral femoral cutaneous nerve, which runs from your spine through your pelvis and upper thigh and supplies feeling to the skin of your thigh. Increased pressure in your groin area can trap this nerve. Possible causes include

- wearing tight pants, stockings, or belts
- weight gain, obesity
- pregnancy
- wearing something heavy (like a tool belt) around your waist or carrying something heavy (such as a wallet or cellphone) in your front or side pants pocket
- scar tissue from a past surgery in your groin area
- nerve damage from diabetes, alcohol abuse, or an accident
- lead poisoning.

About four out of every 100,000 people will develop meralgia paresthetica. This condition is most common in people ages 30 to 40. Meralgia paresthetica has recently earned the nickname "skinny pants syndrome" in reference to the trend among young people of wearing tight, constricting jeans.

### Diagnosing meralgia paresthetica

Meralgia paresthetica is often misdiagnosed because it can mimic other problems such as spinal nerve damage, uterine fibroids, appendicitis, or a tumor. Usually a medical history and physical exam will provide your

### ▶ Symptoms of meralgia paresthetica

- Numbness, tingling or buzzing, or burning pain on the outside of one thigh
- Pain or numbness that gets worse when you stand or walk, and improves when you sit down
- Aching in the groin that may spread to the buttocks

doctor with enough information to diagnose this condition. The doctor may ask you to describe how you feel and what could have happened to trigger nerve compression.

The main method used to diagnose meralgia paresthetica is the pelvic compression test. You lie on your side with the affected leg up. The doctor will press down on the area where the nerve is compressed and hold it for about 45 seconds. If you have the condition, you will feel pain when the doctor presses down. The doctor may also test for numbness by running a brush lightly over the side of your thigh.

Imaging tests such as x-ray, CT, or MRI are not needed to diagnose meralgia paresthetica, but may be recommended to rule out other possible causes of your pain. As examples, an x-ray of your pelvis and hip can identify osteoarthritis of the hip. MRI can rule out a herniated disc or nerve damage. And ultrasound can help determine whether fibroids are the cause in women. Electromyography and nerve conduction studies (see "Nerve studies," page 25) can help diagnose other nerve-related conditions, such as a pinched nerve in the spine.

### Treating meralgia paresthetica

The goal in treating meralgia paresthetica is to relieve pressure on the nerve. You may be able to do this by wearing looser clothing or losing weight. An over-the-counter pain reliever such as ibuprofen or acetaminophen (Tylenol) can help with discomfort in the meantime.

Physical therapy strengthens the leg muscles, improves flexibility, and relieves tension in your lower back and buttocks. One exercise that helps take pressure off the lateral femoral cutaneous nerve is called cat-cow (see Figure 8, at right).

Most people will get better within a few weeks using these treatments. If you need something stronger, your doctor might recommend a tricyclic antidepressant, or an antiseizure medicine such as gabapentin (Neurontin), phenytoin (Dilantin), or pregabalin (Lyrica). These drugs can help ease nerve pain.

Only rarely is surgery necessary to take pressure off the nerve. Surgery for meralgia paresthetica involves removing scar tissue or other restricting tissue around the lateral femoral cutaneous nerve (neurolysis) or cutting out part of the nerve to relieve pressure.

## Sciatica

A sudden, intense pain running down the back of your thigh might feel like a leg injury, but it could actually be a sign of a nerve problem stemming from your lower back. Sciatica isn't a condition itself. Rather, it's a symptom—a radiating pain in your leg that usually

---

### Figure 8: Cat-cow stretch

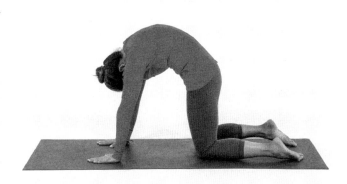

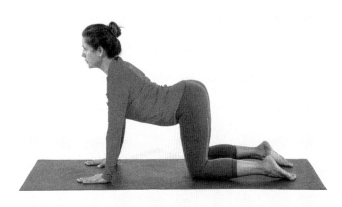

This popular stretch is good for the back, chest, and abdomen. Here's how to do it:

- Get on all fours with your hands placed directly under your shoulders and your knees directly below your hips at a 90° angle.
- Slowly drop your head down and round your back up toward the ceiling. Hold for about 15 seconds. Then return to the starting position.
- Now flex your back in the opposite direction, lifting your chest and head toward the ceiling. Hold this position for about 15 seconds. Repeat the entire sequence three to five times.

occurs when a spinal disc presses on nerve roots in your lower spine.

To understand sciatica, it helps to know a little bit of back anatomy. Your spine is made up of 24 bones called vertebrae. The five vertebrae in the lower back are known collectively as the lumbar spine. In between each vertebra and the one next to it is a flat, round disc filled with a thick, jelly-like substance. These discs act as cushioning between the vertebrae.

The sciatic nerve is formed from several nerves that individually run down your lower back, converge into one nerve in your buttocks, and then stretch down each leg. It's the longest nerve in your body, extending all the way down through each foot and into your toes. Its job is to relay messages to and from your brain, through your spinal cord, to your legs and feet.

Sciatica happens when the roots of the sciatic nerve in your lower back are compressed or squeezed. The most common cause is pressure from a herniated ("slipped") disc. When the outer covering of a disc develops a tear, the insides of the disc can bulge out, similar to what would happen if you were to gently press on a jelly donut. The bulging disc puts pressure on nerve roots around it.

Other possible causes of sciatica include a narrowing of the spinal canal (spinal stenosis), bone injuries, tumors, infections, and pregnancy. Compression may develop gradually over the years, as the result of wear and tear that accumulates with age. Or, it may result from an injury or more rapid damage to the disc. You're most likely to develop sciatica during your 30s, 40s, or 50s.

Though the nerve pressure is centered in your lower back, it radiates down the nerve into your legs. You'll feel the pain in different areas, depending on which nerve root the bulging disc pinches (see Figure 9, below left).

## Diagnosing sciatica

Both patients and doctors have a tendency to use the term "sciatica" to describe any sharp nerve pain in the back of the thigh. But not all pain in this region is caused by pinching of the sciatic nerve. Other causes include arthritis in the joints of the back or a different nerve disease (such as peripheral neuropathy; see page 45). Because treatment of sciatica may differ from treatments for other causes of pain, it's important for your doctor to determine whether or not your symptoms truly come from sciatica.

During your exam, the doctor will ask you what your pain feels like and where you experience it. You might be asked to move in different ways—such as walking on your heels or toes, lying on your back and raising one straight leg, or squatting—so your doctor can assess the source of the pain. These movements will pinpoint weakness or poor reflexes, which can help your doctor determine whether you have a problem with one of the discs in your back and which nerves are involved.

Your doctor may also use imaging or nerve studies.

**Imaging.** An x-ray or an MRI scan can help your doctor see exactly which nerves are compressed, although it won't necessarily add any information that will aid in your treatment, since sciatica is often treated conservatively with rest and exercise.

## Figure 9: Sciatica: Roots of the problem

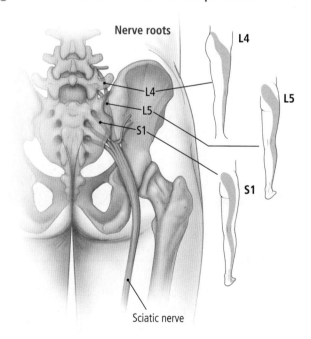

Nerve roots exit from between vertebrae in the spine. At the lower spine, five nerve roots merge to form the sciatic nerve in the leg. If a bulging disc pinches one of these nerve roots, it causes sciatica, sharp pain that typically radiates down the leg. You'll feel the pain in different areas, depending on which nerve root the bulging disc pinches.

### ▶ Symptoms of sciatica

- Lower back pain and a cramping, dull, sharp, throbbing, or shooting pain or a feeling like an electric shock down the back of your leg
- A burning, tingling, or pins-and-needles sensation in the leg
- Increased pain when you move, sit, cough, or sneeze
- Weakness in your legs

**Nerve studies.** Some doctors perform electromyography (EMG) and nerve conduction studies to determine whether there has been any loss in the speed and intensity of nerve signals as they travel through the sciatic nerve. During EMG, the doctor inserts a thin needle into the muscle and records the electrical activity both when the muscle is still and when it is active. During a nerve conduction study, electrodes are placed on the nerve being tested. Then the nerve is stimulated. A computer records the speed and size of nerve impulses to the muscle. Such findings can help confirm the diagnosis and provide more information about where the nerve compression is located.

## Treating sciatica

The pain of sciatica is deceptive. It can be so intense that you think you're dealing with a serious problem that requires surgery. Yet surgery is rarely needed. Sciatica treatment is simple and basic. Rest and time are your two greatest allies. Take it easy, avoiding activities that aggravate your pain, but don't retreat to your bed or couch for hours at a time. Sitting for prolonged periods can actually increase pressure on the discs in your lower back. Gentle movement balanced with short periods of rest are preferable. Try to walk each day. Start with just a few minutes on the treadmill or outside, and gradually lengthen the duration of your walks.

You should also do exercises on your own or with the help of a physical therapist to strengthen your lower back and the abdominal muscles that support it. Gentle stretching can also help. One helpful stretch for sciatica is the single knee pull (see Figure 10, at right).

An over-the-counter anti-inflammatory pain reliever such as aspirin, ibuprofen, or naproxen can make you more comfortable while you heal, as can using a heating pad or cold pack on your lower back or legs for 15 minutes at a time throughout the day. The pain reduction these therapies provide will help you complete the exercises your doctor recommends. Prescription pain medication may be an option for more severe pain, but opioid pain relievers are usually avoided because of the risk of dependence and other side effects. A prescription muscle relaxant such as cyclobenzaprine (Flexeril) may help with muscle spasms, but it may not be recommended for older adults, who can become sedated or confused while on these drugs. If these therapies are not enough, ask your doctor about a corticosteroid injection into your spine.

There's some evidence that acupuncture may be helpful for relieving sciatica pain. Acupuncture has been used in China for more than 3,000 years to treat a variety of medical conditions. Practitioners use hair-thin needles to stimulate various pressure points, which is thought to promote the flow of *qi* (energy) and blood throughout the body. A 2015 review of 12 studies on acupuncture for sciatica found the practice effective for reducing pain, with few side effects (although the authors acknowledged that the overall quality of studies on the subject is poor).

### Figure 10: Single knee pull

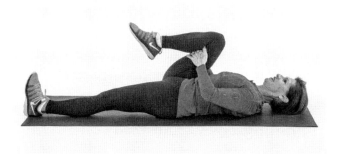

This stretch can help with sciatica. Here's how to do it:
- Lie on your back with your legs straight.
- Raise one knee toward your chest, clasp your hands behind your thigh, and gently pull in.
- Hold the position for 15 to 30 seconds. Repeat with the other leg.
- Repeat the sequence three times, alternating legs.

In up to 90% of people, sciatica will get better with conservative measures within a few weeks. If a herniated disc caused your sciatica, it should improve on its own within three to four months. Rarely is surgery needed to treat a herniated disc, and typically your doctor will recommend it only if you have severe pain that isn't improving, trouble walking, weakness, or a loss of control over your bladder or bowels (a condition known as cauda equina syndrome, a medical emergency) as a result of the compressed nerve. Surgery may also be recommended for a complication known as foot drop, which is difficulty lifting the front part of your foot as you walk. This dragging of the foot results from the nerve injury in your spine, which prevents nerve signals from reaching the muscles needed to lift your foot.

Your pain, and how long you can tolerate it, may ultimately dictate whether you choose surgery. If you can wait it out, you may be able to avoid an operation. After about six to 12 months, people who waited tend to do just as well as those who had surgery.

The surgical procedures used to treat sciatica are known collectively as spinal decompression surgery. There are two types:

- Microdiscectomy is used to remove a herniated disc. It is performed through a small opening in your back. During the procedure, your doctor will remove the damaged part of the disc, along with any loose disc fragments that are putting pressure on your spinal nerve.

- Laminectomy removes the bony plate, called the lamina, covering the back of a vertebra to relieve pressure on the sciatic nerve. Laminectomy may be done at the same time as microdiscectomy.

# Tendinitis

As described in previous chapters, tendons are the thick cords that anchor muscles to bone. Inflammation or irritation of a tendon is known as tendinitis. In the upper leg, tendons in the quadriceps and hamstrings can be affected. The quadriceps tendon attaches the quadriceps muscles to the kneecap (see Figure 11, page 28). It helps to straighten your leg. The three hamstring tendons extend from your pelvis to the top of your lower leg bones. They help you bend your knee and straighten your hip when you run, jump, or kick. Tendinitis can also develop elsewhere in the leg (see page 14 for tendinitis in the hip and page 36 for tendinitis in the knee).

▶ **Symptoms of tendinitis in the upper leg**
- Pain in the lower thigh, above the knee (quadriceps tendinitis)
- Pain in the back of the knee (hamstring tendinitis)
- Swelling or warmth in the affected area

Injuries due to overuse or quick movements (starting, stopping, turning) may cause tendinitis in the upper leg. People who play sports that involve quick acceleration and deceleration, such as soccer, basketball, or volleyball, are most vulnerable to these injuries. Runners can also get tendinitis, especially if they train at high intensity or for long periods of time. Having tight muscles—for example, when you don't adequately warm up before a workout—can increase your risk for this injury. Being obese also makes you more likely to develop tendinitis by putting additional strain on the tendons.

## Diagnosing tendinitis in the upper leg

Your doctor will perform a physical exam, during which he or she will ask about any activities that might have led to the injury. The doctor will then check your range of motion and strength in the affected leg and may order an x-ray to make sure there's no fracture, or MRI to look for inflammation or tears in the tendon.

## Treating tendinitis in the upper leg

Treatment starts by resting the affected leg and taking an anti-inflammatory pain reliever such as aspirin, ibuprofen, or naproxen. A physical therapist can teach you exercises to strengthen and stretch the injured area, and he or she may use additional treatments such as heat, cold, or ultrasound (which delivers heat to the tendon). Wearing a brace (for which the physical therapist can fit you) takes pressure off the tendon, so you can go about your regular activities while it heals. ◤

# Knee pain

The knee isn't the strongest joint in the body—that honor goes to the hip—yet the knee manages to support even more weight, while simultaneously permitting enough flexibility to bend and straighten when you need to sit, stand, kneel, walk, climb stairs, or ride a bicycle. We ask a lot of our knees, which helps explain why they can cause so much trouble.

The knee can be compared to an expensive sports car—a finely tuned machine that is capable of great power but also highly vulnerable to breakdown. Knees suffer more injuries than any other joint, in part because of their complex anatomy and in part because of the demands we place on them. Knee problems can have their roots in a slowly degenerative disease like osteoarthritis, or they can happen as the result of a sudden injury. Overuse injuries can also occur over time. Whatever the cause, knee pain and stiffness can turn the simplest activities, like climbing the stairs or walking to the mailbox, into difficult and painful endeavors.

This chapter explores some of the most common knee ailments (listed in alphabetical order). It begins with an overview of knee anatomy, to explain the different ligaments and other parts of the knee that can cause problems.

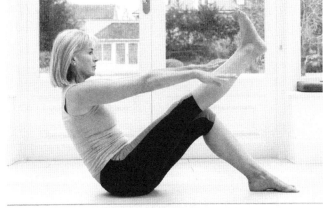

The knee acts as a hinge, but unlike a simple hinge—such as one on a jewelry box or a door, in which any wobble is undesirable—the knee can also slightly rotate or move side to side.

## Knee anatomy 101

The knee joint is a hinge that allows your lower leg and foot to swing easily forward or back as you walk, run, or kick. A healthy knee allows almost 150° of movement. But unlike a simple hinge, the knee can also rotate slightly, thanks to its unique anatomy (see Figure 11, page 28).

### Bones

The knee joint forms at the junction of three bones:
- the thighbone (femur)
- the shin bone (tibia)
- the kneecap (patella).

At the knee, the thighbone divides into two rounded knobs called condyles. These balance on top of the shin bone, which is more or less flat on top with a bump in the middle. In contrast to the perfectly contoured fit between bones in the hip and many other joints, the knee's mismatch in shape allows for complex movement but is quite unstable, like two doorknobs balanced on an uneven plate.

The kneecap is a small bone in the front of the knee. By serving as the attachment point for the quadriceps tendon above the knee and the patellar tendon below the knee (see below), it helps provide leverage for straightening your knee. It sits in a small hollow called the trochlear groove, which is between the two condyles of the thighbone. Whenever you bend and straighten your knee, the kneecap slides up and down inside this groove.

### Ligaments and tendons

Because the thighbone and shin bone do not fit neatly together, ligaments play an especially important role in the knee. Four ligaments running alongside and through the knee create stability and prevent the knee from moving in ways that could damage it.
- The medial collateral ligament (MCL) connects the thighbone to the shin bone on the inside (big-toe

side) of the knee joint, limiting sideways motion.

- The lateral collateral ligament (LCL) does the same thing on the outside (little-toe side) of the knee, but it connects to the fibula instead of the shin bone.
- The anterior cruciate ligament (ACL), located deep within the joint, connects the thighbone to the shin bone in the center of the knee; it keeps the knee from rotating too far or letting your shin get out in front of your thighbone. ACL injuries occur when a sudden stop or turn tears the ligament (see "Ligament injuries," page 30).
- The posterior cruciate ligament (PCL) helps keep the shin bone in place. It crosses behind the ACL, and the two form an *X* in the center of the knee.

In addition, the patellar tendon—actually a ligament, despite its name—connects the kneecap to the shin bone. At the top of the patella, the quadriceps tendon connects the quadriceps muscle to the kneecap and provides the power to extend the leg.

## Cartilage

Knees have two types of cartilage:

- Articular cartilage coats the ends of the bones, enabling the joint to move smoothly.
- Rubbery cartilage pads, each known as a meniscus (plural, menisci), act as shock absorbers between the thighbone and shin bone. These rubbery pads are wedge-shaped—thick on the outer edge and thin on the inside. You have two of them in each knee: the medial meniscus on the inside of the knee joint, and the lateral meniscus on the outside. For their small size, the menisci take a lot of pounding. The medial meniscus carries up to 50% of the load put on the inside of the knee, while the lateral meniscus absorbs about 80% of the force applied to the outside of the knee.

Arthritis of the knee usually involves the degeneration of both types of cartilage. Excess body weight can accelerate degenerative changes in the knee.

---

## Figure 11: The knee: Strong and flexible

### Front view of knee

Anterior cruciate ligament: Connects the femur to the tibia and limits rotation and forward motion of the tibia

Femur (thighbone)

Patella (kneecap)

Posterior cruciate ligament: Crosses behind the ACL and keeps the shin bone in place

Condyle

Condyle

Lateral collateral ligament: Connects the femur to the small bone of the calf (fibula)

Medial collateral ligament: Connects the femur to the tibia, limiting sideways motion

Tibia (shin bone)

Menisci: Shock-absorbing cartilage

Fibula

### Three-quarter view of knee

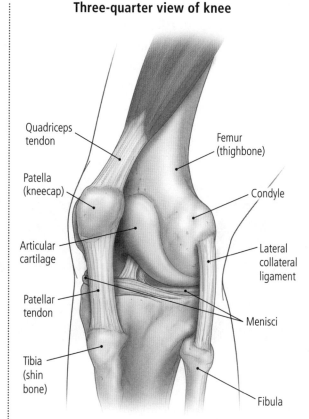

Quadriceps tendon

Patella (kneecap)

Articular cartilage

Patellar tendon

Tibia (shin bone)

Femur (thighbone)

Condyle

Lateral collateral ligament

Menisci

Fibula

The knee joint forms at the junction of the femur, tibia, and patella. Ligaments connect these bones and prevent the knee from moving in a way that could cause damage. The patellar tendon (actually a ligament) attaches the bottom of the patella to the top of the tibia. Two bony protuberances of the femur, called condyles, perch atop the shin bone. Articular cartilage coats the ends of these bones, enabling them to move smoothly against one another. Tendons give the knee stability.

## Bursae

Fluid-filled pouches called bursae act as cushions to prevent bones and soft tissues—muscles, tendons, and skin—from rubbing against one another. All told, the body has 150 bursae, including in the hips, knees, shoulders, and other joints. The knee contains a number of bursae, including the following:

- the prepatellar bursa, between the kneecap and the skin
- the deep infrapatellar bursa, between the patellar tendon and the tibia
- the pes anserine bursa, between the semimembranosus hamstring muscle and the tibia.

Inflammation of these pillow-like sacs results in the painful condition known as bursitis (see "Bursitis," below right).

# Baker's cyst

When a lump appears behind your knee, it can be disconcerting at the very least, if not alarming. But if the lump is a Baker's cyst, you can rest easy knowing that you have a benign condition that is relatively simple to relieve. A Baker's cyst (also called a popliteal cyst) is a fluid-filled sac, or cyst, that forms when the knee produces too much synovial fluid (the viscous liquid that lubricates this joint and prevents friction). Arthritis or an injury such as a tear in the cartilage or a meniscus can ramp up synovial fluid production. Baker's cysts are named for William Morrant Baker, the 19th-century surgeon who described the condition in eight of his patients. In Baker's era, treatment sometimes involved amputation. Today, much less radical measures are used.

Although this condition isn't serious, any swelling behind your knee should prompt a call to your doctor. There is a small chance that an unusual growth or fluid collection indicates an infection, aneurysm, blood clot, or other serious condition.

### Diagnosing Baker's cyst

Sometimes your symptoms alone will reveal the cause of the lump. You may need an imaging test such as ultrasound or MRI to confirm that you don't have a blood clot or another serious condition.

▶ **Symptoms of Baker's cyst**

- A soft lump behind your knee
- Pain in your knee
- Stiffness
- Difficulty fully bending your knee
- Swelling in one leg

### Treating Baker's cyst

Some cysts will gradually disappear on their own or burst, in which case your body will reabsorb the fluid. Resting and elevating the leg as well as holding an ice pack to the back of your knee will help control inflammation. A corticosteroid shot can sometimes shrink the cyst more quickly. If the cyst doesn't go away, your doctor can drain the fluid with a needle (a procedure called needle aspiration). In addition to managing symptoms with these measures, you'll need to treat the cause of the cyst. Anti-inflammatory or pain medicines (see "Treating knee osteoarthritis," page 34) or surgery to repair torn cartilage (see "Treating meniscal tears," page 32) can prevent the problem from recurring.

# Bursitis

Bursae are the pillow-like pouches that act as cushions between bones and soft tissues. There are 11 bursae in and around the knee. When any one of them becomes inflamed because of an injury, excessive pressure, or other causes, that is called bursitis. These are the three most common types of knee bursitis:

- Prepatellar bursitis—nicknamed "housemaid's knee" or "clergyman's knee"—affects the bursa between the kneecap and your skin, causing swelling on top of or in front of the kneecap. It is common among people whose jobs or hobbies require a lot of kneeling, such as plumbers, roofers, gardeners, and housecleaners.
- Infrapatellar bursitis affects the bursa just below the kneecap. It is also common in people who spend a lot of time kneeling.
- Pes anserine bursitis affects the bursa between your shin bone and the hamstring tendons. It is more often seen in runners.

## ▶ Symptoms of knee bursitis

**For prepatellar or infrapatellar bursitis:**

- Swelling on top of the kneecap (prepatellar bursitis) or below the kneecap (infrapatellar bursitis)
- Warmth and tenderness
- Pain when you move, rest, or kneel

**For pes anserine bursitis:**

- Pain located inside the knee, below the knee joint
- An increase in pain when you climb stairs or exercise
- Pain when your knees touch as you lie on your side

## Diagnosing knee bursitis

Your doctor will examine your knees, looking for warmth, redness, and pain. Imaging tests such as MRI or ultrasound can show if there is any swelling in the knee bursae.

## Treating knee bursitis

Bursitis often gets better on its own, once you stop doing the activity that caused it. Follow the RICE protocol: rest, ice, compression, and elevation (see "Treating a hamstring strain or tear," page 19). Take an over-the-counter anti-inflammatory pain reliever—such as aspirin, ibuprofen (Advil, Motrin), or naproxen (Aleve)—to reduce swelling and pain. A physical therapist can work with you to increase flexibility and strengthen the muscles that support your knee. If the cause is an infection, an antibiotic should clear it up. For more stubborn swelling, you might try a corticosteroid injection or aspiration to remove excess fluid from the knee. If bursitis doesn't improve, your doctor might recommend surgery to remove the inflamed bursa.

To prevent knee bursitis in the future, avoid kneeling on hard surfaces for any length of time. If you do have to kneel, use a cushion or knee pads for protection.

## Ligament injuries (sprains)

A sprain (stretching or tearing) of any of the knee's four ligaments (see Figure 11, page 28) can destabilize the joint and make it difficult to turn or twist the leg.

The ACL is the most commonly injured knee ligament. The ACL can stretch or tear during any sudden movement in which your feet stay in place while your knees twist, which often happens in sports like skiing, football, soccer, or basketball. Female athletes are two to eight times more likely to tear an ACL than male athletes. One factor is female anatomy. Because women have wider hips relative to their body size, the thighbone slants inward toward the knee at a steeper angle than in men (see Figure 12, page 31), placing additional stress on this ligament and making it more vulnerable to tearing.

The PCL in the back of the knee is also commonly injured. Because of the PCL's more protected location, tearing it usually requires a hard blow, for example, from a football tackle or a car crash.

The two collateral ligaments give stability to the inner and outer knee. The MCL and LCL can be torn by a hit to the inner or outer side of the knee, which may occur in sports like football or hockey. Because of the way the knee joint is structured, an injury of the LCL will usually occur along with damage to other structures of the joint, such as the ACL or a meniscus.

## Diagnosing ligament injuries

Your doctor will ask about the injury and then examine your knee, looking for areas of tenderness, instability, limited range of motion, and buckling when you walk. The location of the pain and buckling can help your doctor pinpoint which ligament you have injured. For example, in an MCL sprain the knee will buckle toward the outside. If the exam indicates a ligament injury, you may get an imaging test such as an

### Sprains and strains: What's the difference?

Sprains and strains are easy to confuse since only one letter separates these two conditions, but they are not the same.

- A sprain is a stretch or tear in a ligament. In the case of the knees, that means one of the four knee ligaments (see "Ligament injuries," at left).
- A strain is a stretch or tear in a muscle or tendon. In the knee, that would be a muscle or tendon supporting the knee (see "Strains," page 36).

x-ray or MRI to look for tears and other damage to the joint. Doctors grade ligament sprains as follows:

- **Grade 1** sprains occur when the ligament stretches, but not to the point where the knee becomes destabilized.
- **Grade 2** sprains, or partial tears, happen when the ligament is stretched enough to loosen, or destabilize, the joint.
- **Grade 3** sprains, or complete tears, occur when the ligament rips and cannot support the joint.

### Treating ligament injuries

As with other injuries, rest, ice, compression, and elevation (RICE) is the primary treatment (see "Treating a hamstring strain or tear," page 19). Over-the-counter anti-inflammatory pain relievers can be helpful for bringing down swelling. Your doctor will recommend that you sit out sports or exercise until the knee heals and wear a protective knee brace when you do play again. Physical therapy will help strengthen the muscles that support your knee. Most mild (grade 1 or 2) sprains heal within two to four weeks, but more severe tears take up to a year to fully heal, and they may require surgery.

### ▷ Symptoms of ligament injuries

**For injury to the anterior cruciate ligament (ACL):**

- A popping sound when the injury happens
- Swelling, which may cause pain
- Difficulty standing on the affected knee, or a feeling like your knee is giving way

**For injury to the posterior cruciate ligament (PCL):**

- Mild to moderate pain that may cause a slight limp or difficulty walking
- Swelling in the knee
- Instability in the knee, which may feel as if it's going to give way

**For injury to the medial collateral ligament (MCL):**

- Pain and tenderness on the inside of the knee
- Wobbling of the knee or the knee giving way
- Swelling
- Sensation of "opening up" with each step (in severe injuries)

A knee ligament that is completely torn makes it difficult to twist or turn the knee. The joint may become too weak to support your weight, causing it to give way or buckle. If this happens, you may need ligament repair surgery. During this procedure, the surgeon will take a piece of tendon from your knee-cap, hamstring, or quadriceps (called an autograft) or from a donor (called an allograft) and attach it to your thighbone and shin bone to hold the knee joint together and support it. Often this is done arthroscopically, through small incisions.

## Meniscal tears

The knee comes equipped with two built-in shock absorbers between the shin bone and thighbone—crescent-shaped pads of cartilage called the medial meniscus and the lateral meniscus (plural, menisci). Although thick and rubbery, the menisci can rip if

---

### Figure 12: What's your Q-angle?

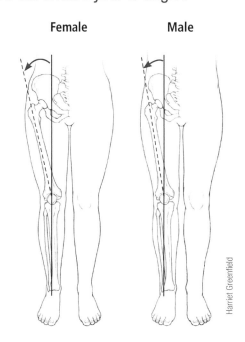

Female          Male

It's not obvious, but your thighbone (femur) and your shin bone (tibia) are not positioned in a straight line. The line of the femur and the line extending from the ankle through the kneecap (patella) form what is known as the Q-angle. Women usually have a more pronounced Q-angle than men. Because a greater Q-angle is associated with a higher incidence of tears in the anterior cruciate ligament (ACL), women are more susceptible to these tears.

exposed to enough force, such as from a football tackle or by twisting the knee while skiing or dancing.

Meniscal tears (see Figure 13, below) are among the most common knee injuries, particularly in athletes who play football and other contact sports. Older adults are also prone to these tears, as cartilage of the knee wears away over time and leaves the joint more vulnerable. In an older adult, a simple twist of the knee can tear an already weakened meniscus. Such injuries are called degenerative meniscal tears.

Doctors classify meniscal tears by their location, pattern, and severity. Each meniscus has three zones—the anterior horn (at the front), the body (in the middle), and the posterior horn (at the back). Tears can occur in any of these three areas. The posterior horn is the thickest and most weightbearing part of the meniscus, and the most common location for tears.

Meniscal tears come in a variety of patterns. Their names are often colorful ways of describing their shapes. For example, a bucket-handle tear describes an injury in which part of the meniscus rips and flips over, forming an upside-down *U* shape like the handle on a bucket. A parrot-beak tear cuts through the meniscus, producing a curved cut-out that resembles the hooked shape of that bird's beak. A horizontal tear

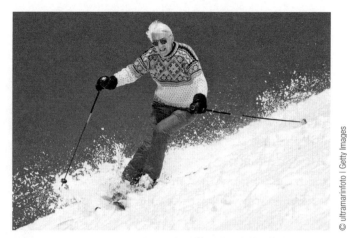

Skiing is among the sports that pose a risk of meniscal tears. A small tear on the outer edge of the meniscus may not need treatment, since the outer third has an ample blood supply.

runs in a straight line across the lower portion of the meniscus. Tears that encompass more than one type are called complex tears.

## Diagnosing meniscal tears

After asking about your symptoms and the activities that preceded them, your doctor will feel your knee joint for pain and swelling. One way to check for a meniscal tear is with the McMurray test. Your doctor will bend, straighten, and rotate your knee. A clicking sound heard during these movements can indicate a meniscal tear. MRI can help your doctor visualize the tear, while an x-ray helps to rule out osteoarthritis and other bone-related causes of knee pain.

## Treating meniscal tears

Where a tear occurs and how large it is will dictate how it is treated.

## ▶ Symptoms of a meniscal tear

- A popping sensation
- Swelling and stiffness that increases in the day or so after the injury
- Pain that gets worse when you twist or bend the knee
- A feeling that the knee is catching or locking when you walk
- Difficulty fully straightening your knee
- Weakness and reduced range of motion in the knee

## Figure 13: Torn meniscus

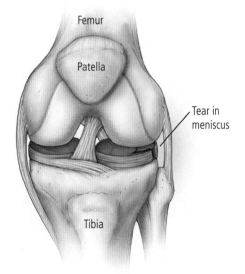

Femur

Patella

Tear in meniscus

Tibia

When the shock-absorbing cartilage in the knee is torn by injury or worn ragged by use, the result is a torn meniscus. Stiffness and a sensation that the knee is catching or locking often result.

Small tears on the outer edge of the meniscus may not need treatment, unless they cause excessive pain or instability, since the outer third of the meniscus has an ample blood supply that can help the wound heal. Follow the RICE (rest, ice, compression, elevation) protocol, and take an over-the-counter anti-inflammatory pain reliever such as aspirin, ibuprofen, or naproxen to manage pain and swelling. These measures may have a noticeable effect in four to six weeks.

Tears in the center of the meniscus or large tears, however, will not heal on their own. For these tears, arthroscopic surgery may be an option. Through tiny incisions, using a miniature camera and small instruments, the surgeon will trim away the damaged meniscus tissue (partial meniscectomy) or reattach the torn pieces with sutures (meniscus repair). If the knee is completely locked (unable to bend or straighten), surgery must be done right away to remove the section of torn meniscus that is trapped and blocking movement of the knee. After meniscus repair surgery, you will need about three months of rehabilitation to regain strength and function in your knee.

# Osteoarthritis

Arthritis is a collection of diseases that cause pain, swelling, and stiffness in the joints. The most common of these is osteoarthritis. Although osteoarthritis can appear in any joint, the knee is particularly vulnerable, in part because it repeatedly bears almost all the body's weight and partly because it is also subject to sudden injuries, such as meniscal tears (see page 31).

Arthritis is not unique to the modern era. Skeletons of prehistoric hunter-gatherers unearthed by archaeologists show signs of arthritis in their knee joints. But the condition is on the increase. Since the middle of the 20th century, arthritis has doubled in prevalence, in part because of preventable risk factors like weight gain and certain types of sports injuries. The average age at which knee osteoarthritis strikes has dropped from 69 to 56 since the 1990s.

Whatever the cause, the result is pain and disability. Early in the course of the disease, the space between your thighbone and shin bone decreases as the cartilage wears away (see Figure 14, below). Once the cartilage disappears, bone rubs on bone, causing stiffness, an aching pain, or occasional flares of intense pain, and often the formation of bony growths known as bone spurs (osteophytes) around the joint.

## Diagnosing knee osteoarthritis

Your doctor will ask about your symptoms and will look for signs of arthritis like swelling, warmth, redness, loss of motion, or a crackling sound (crepitus) when you bend and straighten the knee. An x-ray can reveal narrowing in the joint space, as well as abnor-

▷ **Symptoms of knee osteoarthritis**

- Stiffness and swelling in one or both knees
- Warmth and redness in the joint
- Pain that gets worse with use or if you sit for a long period of time
- A cracking, popping, or sticking sound when you move the knee
- Weakness in the knee

## Figure 14: Knee osteoarthritis

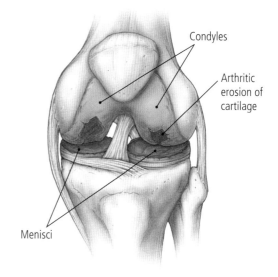

Condyles

Arthritic erosion of cartilage

Menisci

Age, mechanical wear and tear, genetics, and biochemical factors all contribute to the gradual degeneration of the cartilage and the meniscus. In this illustration, articular cartilage in the knee has worn down and eroded. Tenderness, stiffness, and morning pain are tell-tale signs of osteoarthritis.

## Figure 15: Total knee replacement surgery

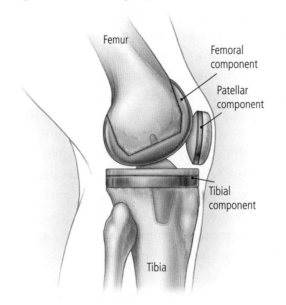

The surgeon first cuts away thin slices of bone with damaged cartilage from the end of the thighbone (femur) and the top of the shin bone (tibia), making sure that the bones are cut to precisely fit the shape of the replacement pieces. The artificial joint is attached to the bones with cement or screws. A small plastic piece goes on the back of the kneecap (patella) to ride smoothly over the other parts of the artificial joint when you bend your knee.

Femur

Femoral component

Patellar component

Tibial component

Tibia

mal bony outgrowths (bone spurs) caused by joint damage. If your doctor suspects rheumatoid arthritis, you may have blood tests for signs of inflammation and autoantibodies. If gout (another form of arthritis) is a possibility, you may be tested for elevated uric acid.

### Treating knee osteoarthritis

Osteoarthritis has no cure, so doctors focus on three things when treating the condition: relieving pain, protecting joints from further damage, and improving muscle tone to help stabilize joints. Losing weight if you are overweight or obese is essential to getting knee osteoarthritis under control. With each step you take, you put one-and-a-half times the force of your body weight onto your knees. Climb stairs, and the force on your knees will reach double that of your body weight. Increasing your physical activity level and changing your diet can help you get to your desired weight.

For pain relief, over-the-counter nonsteroidal anti-inflammatory drugs (NSAIDs)—such as aspirin, ibuprofen, or naproxen—play an important role. However, NSAIDs may cause stomach bleeding or other side effects. Acetaminophen (Tylenol) is easier on the stomach, but it may be less effective for osteoarthritis; if you take it, be sure not to exceed the maximum dosage of 3,000 milligrams per day. Some of these drugs also come in rub-on versions that avoid

some of the bodywide side effects of the oral drugs.

To relieve more severe pain, your doctor might recommend injections of corticosteroids or hyaluronic acid (a lubricating fluid that is naturally found in healthy joints). Supplements containing glucosamine and chondroitin sulfate (substances found naturally in cartilage) are often touted for promoting joint pain relief, but there is no real evidence they help with knee arthritis.

Pain relievers, however, are only part of the solution. To help strengthen the supporting muscles around the knee, your doctor will likely prescribe physical therapy. A physical therapist helps you restore and maintain function, usually with an exercise program that is individually tailored to your needs. The therapist may also apply ultrasound, heat or cold, or a variety of other therapies to help relieve pain. He or she may also educate you about posture and body mechanics and suggest assistive devices to help protect your knees.

Assistive devices can help you get around more easily when your knees are sore. Placing special insoles into your shoes redistributes your weight, shifting the load off your knees. An unloader brace also moves weight off the painful part of the knee. A cane or walker can be invaluable for helping you get around without falling (see "Finding the assistive device that fits you," page 12).

If you've tried a number of treatments and are still dealing with debilitatingly stiff, achy knees, your doctor might suggest one of these surgical procedures:

**Cartilage grafting** removes a piece of healthy cartilage from another part of your body and uses it to plug a small area of damaged cartilage in your knee. This procedure is best suited to younger people who have minimal cartilage damage.

**Osteotomy** takes a small piece of bone from either the tibia or femur and uses it as a bolster to shift your weight off the damaged part of your knee.

**Total or partial knee replacement** removes damaged cartilage and bone and replaces them with an artificial metal or plastic joint or components (see Figure 15, page 34).

# Patellofemoral pain syndrome

Patellofemoral pain syndrome is a catchall term for pain around the kneecap (patella) that's caused by a variety of factors. Inflammation and pain in this area is sometimes referred to as "runner's knee," but it can also occur during non-athletic activities. About 22% of people over all, and 29% of teenagers, develop this condition each year. Patellofemoral pain syndrome is the leading cause of knee pain in female athletes.

Although the syndrome may have any of several causes (including tendinitis in the knee; see page 36), the term frequently refers to pain stemming from a misalignment in the kneecap. Instead of moving back and forth inside the trochlear groove when the knee bends, the patella moves out to one side of the groove, which increases pressure on the soft tissues of the knee. This abnormal movement may be caused by muscle weakness, tightness, or imbalance; a larger-than-normal Q-angle (see Figure 12, page 31); or an overly tight tendon that pulls the patella out of place.

Overuse—for example, from running or climbing stairs frequently—is one of the most common causes. Suddenly jacking up your workouts or using the wrong technique can also lead to pain. Repeatedly bending and straightening your knee increases pressure between the patella and femur, and it irritates the patella. Damage to the tendons, cartilage, or bones of the knee can also contribute to this condition.

## ▶ Symptoms of patellofemoral pain syndrome

- Dull, aching pain in the front of the knee, especially during activities like running, climbing stairs, jumping, kneeling, or squatting
- Pain when you get up after sitting for several hours with your knees bent, such as on a long airplane trip
- Popping or crackling sounds when you move your knee

## Diagnosing patellofemoral pain syndrome

During the exam, your doctor will ask what you've been doing that might have triggered knee pain and what activities make the pain worse. The doctor will gently press on your knee to identify areas of tenderness and will look at your leg and knee alignment, strength, and flexibility while you bend and straighten the joint. You may be asked to move in different ways—for example, walking, squatting, or lunging—so the doctor can assess your knee and leg strength and look for any changes in your gait. An x-ray can help rule out arthritis or other bone problems, while an MRI or CT scan will reveal any cartilage loss, ligament problems, and meniscal tears.

## Treating patellofemoral pain syndrome

The treatment your doctor recommends depends on the cause of your knee pain. You'll want to take a break from the activity that caused the pain. Rather than jogging or climbing stairs, do non-impact exercises like biking or swimming to avoid putting pressure on your knee. Use the RICE (rest, ice, compression, elevation) method to give your knee time to recover (see "Treating a hamstring strain or tear," page 19). Take an over-the-counter anti-inflammatory pain reliever such as aspirin, ibuprofen, or naproxen to bring down swelling and ease your pain. Exercises to strengthen your quadriceps, hamstrings, and core muscles will provide more stability to your knee. You can do these exercises on your own or with a physical therapist.

Your doctor might also recommend wearing orthotics, special shoe inserts that put your leg into better alignment to take pressure off your knee. You can buy these inserts over the counter or have them specially ordered for you at your doctor's office. A knee brace or taping will help stabilize the painful joint whenever you exercise or participate in sports. It can take six weeks or more to notice an improvement, but it's important to see your therapy through to the end. Inadequate treatment is one reason why more than half of people with patellofemoral pain syndrome still complain of pain five or more years after they are first diagnosed.

Surgery is rarely needed unless your pain is severe and it does not improve with conservative treatments.

Doctors can remove damaged cartilage and bone from the surface of the kneecap or adjust tendons to correct the misalignment arthroscopically (through small incisions).

## Strains

A knee strain is a stretch or tear in a muscle or tendon that supports the knee. It is typically caused by an accident such as a fall or twisting motion that stretches the tissues of the joints past their limits. Strains are common among people who play football and other contact sports, but they can also occur as the result of poor form, overuse, tight or weak muscles, or wearing the wrong footwear.

### Diagnosing knee strain

Distinguishing sprains from strains may be challenging because of the number and complexity of structures that make up your knee (see "Sprains and strains: What's the difference?" on page 30). Your doctor will use your symptoms and a description of the injury that caused them as a guide to pinpoint which of the two problems you have. Strains are graded in much the same way as sprains, and the grade of your injury can help determine which treatment you need (see "Diagnosing ligament injuries," page 30). MRI may aid in the diagnosis by revealing tears in muscles, ligaments, or cartilage.

### Treating knee strain

Most people can self-treat knee strains with the RICE (rest, ice, compression, elevation) method. Wearing a brace on your knee will help support the injured joint while it heals. After an injury, it's common for the knee to become stiff and difficult to move. Doing exercises with a physical therapist will help strengthen the joint and restore full range of motion. Mild strains should heal within six weeks. It may take more than four months for a more severe tear to heal, and some will require surgery to fix. Most of these procedures are done arthroscopically, through small incisions using tiny instruments.

## Tendinitis

Tendinitis is inflammation in a tendon. In the case of the knee, the damage typically occurs to the patellar tendon, the bridge between your kneecap (patella) and shin bone (tibia). Patellar tendon disease or inflammation is sometimes referred to as "jumper's knee," because athletes in sports that involve a lot of jumping on hard surfaces, such as basketball and volleyball, are more likely to develop this injury.

Repeated stress from the weight of your body while running or jumping may cause inflammation and tiny tears to form in the patellar tendon. As the number of tears increases, the tendon progressively weakens and becomes more painful. You are more likely to develop knee tendinitis if you have tight thigh muscles or an imbalance of stronger to weaker muscles in your knees, both of which can increase pressure on your patellar tendon.

The quadriceps tendon can also be injured, but this is not as common.

### Diagnosing tendinitis in the knee

After asking about your symptoms and any activities that might have caused this injury, your doctor will gently press on your knee to see where the pain is centered. Discomfort just below your kneecap is a sign of tendinitis. You may need an x-ray to see if your

> ### Symptoms of knee strain
> - A popping noise when the injury occurs
> - Pain
> - Stiffness
> - Swelling
> - Bruising
> - Weakness

> ### Symptoms of tendinitis in the knee
> - Pain and tenderness in the front of your knee, just below your kneecap
> - Pain when you walk, run, or jump, which may improve when you rest
> - Swelling
> - A cracking sound when you move the knee

pain stems from a bone or joint problem in the knee. Ultrasound or MRI can reveal tears or other damage in your patellar tendon.

## Treating tendinitis in the knee

Ice, rest, and over-the-counter pain relievers can help you manage discomfort in your knee until it heals. In the meantime, a physical therapist can teach you exer-cises to stretch and lengthen the muscles of your knee, and to strengthen these muscles to take pressure off your patellar tendon. One exercise that's often recom-mended for patellar tendinitis is the eccentric drop squat, which involves rapidly dropping into a quarter-squat (but don't drop lower than that) and then slowly standing back up. Another is the straight-leg raise (see Figure 16, at left). Your physical therapist might recommend an orthotic device called a patellar ten-don strap, which applies compression to your tendon to redistribute some of the pressure off of it and onto other parts of your knee.

If these measures don't work, a corticosteroid injection in the knee can help relieve pain. A newer treatment injects the sugar dextrose into the knee. Dextrose acts as an irritant, which is believed to stim-ulate collagen growth and connective tissue repair. However, its overall effectiveness is uncertain. Plate-let-rich plasma (PRP) injection (see "Treating a ham-string strain or tear," page 19) is also being investigated as a treatment for knee tendinitis. Early studies show promise, but the research is still preliminary.

Tendinitis should improve within a few weeks. Your doctor will likely recommend taking a break from whatever activity caused the injury until the tendon heals. If you don't see any improvement, your doctor might recommend arthroscopic surgery to remove damaged tissue from the knee (a procedure called debridement). ◥

---

## Figure 16: Straight-leg raise

Strong muscles around a damaged knee can help support the joint. For example, a strong quadriceps can take over the shock-absorbing role usually played by the meniscus or cartilage in the knee. This exercise, called a straight-leg raise, helps strengthen the quadriceps.

To do this exercise:

- Lie on your back with your legs outstretched in front of you. Bend one knee into a 90° angle, keeping your foot on the floor.

- In this position, slowly lift the other leg about six to 12 inches off the floor. Hold for 10 seconds. Slowly lower your leg.

- Repeat until your thigh feels fatigued, then switch to the other leg.

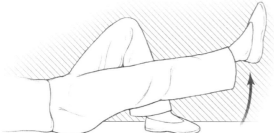

# Lower leg pain

Your lower legs take a lot of wear and tear. Despite their comparatively small size in relation to your upper legs, they carry a greater weight, and they must contend with the difficult job of pumping blood back up toward the heart. The sources of pain in your lower legs can range from muscle and tendon issues to blood vessel problems and skin sores. This chapter elaborates on some of the main problems that can affect your calves and shins (listed in alphabetical order). It starts with a look at the anatomy of the lower leg.

## Lower leg anatomy 101

Bones, muscles, tendons, and blood vessels in the lower leg have a lot in common with their counterparts in the upper leg, yet their position near the body's extremities poses some additional challenges.

### Bones

The lower leg has just two bones.

**The tibia (shin bone)** is the larger of the two bones in the lower leg. It is actually the second largest bone in the body (only the thighbone is bigger) and the one that supports most of your weight. It connects to the thighbone at the knee, and to the bones of the foot at the ankle joint.

**The fibula (calf bone)** runs parallel to the shin bone, but it is thinner and weaker. Whereas you can easily feel the shin bone by running your hand down the front of your lower leg, you may not even be aware of the existence of the calf bone. Still, it provides essential stability for the shin bone.

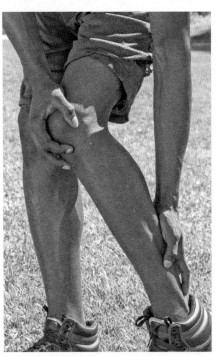

The Achilles tendon is the thick, fibrous band of tissue that connects your calf muscles to your ankle. Achilles tendinitis is a common affliction among runners.

### Muscles

Muscles in the lower leg are integral to movements of the ankle, foot, and toes.

**Gastrocnemius.** The main calf muscle (gastrocnemius) is the largest muscle in the back of the lower leg, and the one that bulges out if you regularly strengthen your calves by bike riding or climbing stairs. This diamond-shaped muscle begins at the bottom of the femur and attaches to the Achilles tendon at the heel. It allows you to extend your foot downward, as well as to run and jump.

**Soleus.** Underneath the gastrocnemius is a smaller, flatter muscle called the soleus, which pulls tightly to help your body remain upright. You also use this muscle whenever you walk or run.

**Plantaris.** In between the gastrocnemius and soleus is a pencil-thin muscle called the plantaris that works with the Achilles tendon to allow you to rise up onto your toes or point your foot. Interestingly enough, 10% to 20% of people are born without a plantaris muscle. In those who lack a plantaris muscle, the gastrocnemius takes over its work.

### Tendons

The Achilles tendon attaches all three muscles in the lower leg—the gastrocnemius, plantaris, and soleus—to the heel bone. It is the main connection point between the leg and foot, and it gives you the ability to run and jump. Because the structures of the legs and feet are so closely connected, a problem with one can lead to problems with the other. For example, when your feet hurt, you may adapt the way you walk to avoid discomfort. Changing your gait alters the mechanics of your ankle joint, which can lead to ankle pain. Pain in your ankle makes you adjust your leg movements, which can potentially lead to knee or hip issues. Continuing to move in an unnatural way can contribute to ongoing pain.

## Blood vessels

As in the rest of the body, the arteries deliver blood from the heart, and the veins ferry it back. But arteries in the lower leg are particularly vulnerable to circulation problems (see "Peripheral artery disease and claudication," page 43), and the hydraulic challenge of pumping blood upward is greatest in the lower legs (see "Edema," page 41).

# Achilles tendinitis and tendon tear

The Achilles tendon is the thick, fibrous band of tissue that runs down the back of your lower leg. It connects your calf muscles to your heel and helps you run, jump, and walk. This tendon, the largest in your body, gets its name from Achilles, the mythological Greek hero of the Trojan war. Achilles was exceptionally strong, but he had one vulnerability—a tiny area on his heel where his mother had held him while dipping him into the river Styx to make him invincible. If you play sports frequently enough to injure this tendon, it could turn into your own "Achilles' heel," causing pain and inflammation severe enough to limit your activities.

Achilles tendinitis primarily affects people who overwork this tendon when they run, walk, or jump excessively. This is a common affliction among runners, particularly if they suddenly increase the intensity or duration of their training sessions or frequently run up hills. Some 66% of joggers complain of pain in their Achilles tendon at one time or another. Repetitive stress causes fibers in the Achilles tendon to break down, making the tendon swell. However, you don't need to be an athlete to develop Achilles tendinitis. Age also weakens this structure and makes it more prone to strain or tears. Certain physical characteristics, including flat feet and tight calf muscles, also increase the likelihood of tendinitis.

▶ **Symptoms of Achilles tendinitis**
- Pain in the back of the lower leg, just above the heel, that gets worse after long periods of running, walking, or stair climbing
- Swelling
- Stiffness that may improve with activity
- Reduced range of motion, especially difficulty flexing your foot or standing up on your toes

▶ **Symptoms of Achilles tendon tear**
- A popping sound
- Swelling
- Sudden pain in the heel

Achilles tendinitis is divided into two types, based on the part of the tendon that is inflamed:
- Non-insertional Achilles tendinitis affects fibers in the center of the tendon. This type is more common among young, active people.
- Insertional Achilles tendinitis affects the bottom of the heel, in the spot where the tendon attaches (the technical term is "inserts") into the heel bone. An abnormal piece of extra bone, called a bone spur (osteophyte), may also grow on the heel. This type of tendinitis can affect people of any age, but it often occurs after years of running or other overuse.

Tendon weakness—or an injury from too much force on the heel—can also rip the Achilles tendon. This is known as a tendon rupture or tear. You'll know your tendon has ruptured by signs like a popping sound, swelling, and sudden pain in the heel. If you hear that telltale popping sound, get medical help right away. Waiting too long to see a doctor can make surgical repair more difficult if you ultimately need it.

## Diagnosing Achilles tendinitis and tendon tear

Your doctor will ask about your symptoms and activities before examining the back of your heel to look for swelling, pain, and thickening of the Achilles tendon. You may be asked to stand on your toes. An inability to do so is a sign you've injured this tendon.

To determine whether you've ruptured your tendon, your doctor may do the Thompson test. You'll lie face down with your feet hanging off the end of the table. When the doctor squeezes your calf muscle, your big toe should flex. A lack of movement indicates a tendon rupture.

In addition to the exam, your doctor might send you for x-rays to look for calcium deposits where the tendon attaches to the heel (indicating calcific tendinitis) or an MRI scan to reveal the severity of damage to the tendon. Knowing how badly the tendon is injured can help your doctor plan surgery, if needed.

## Treating Achilles tendinitis and tendon tear

The first step in treatment is to stop the activity that caused your Achilles tendinitis. Avoid high-impact exercises such as running or stair climbing that put pressure on the tendon. Switch to non-impact exercises like biking, swimming, and elliptical training. Use an ice pack on the affected tendon for 15 to 20 minutes at a time, a few times a day. (Never place ice directly on the skin. Place a thin towel between your skin and the ice pack.) An over-the counter pain reliever such as aspirin, ibuprofen (Advil, Motrin), or naproxen (Aleve) can also help reduce swelling and pain.

Physical therapy is an effective treatment, especially for non-insertional tendinitis. The therapist will teach you exercises to strengthen muscles around the heel. One specific program used to treat Achilles tendinitis is called eccentric training, or the Alfredson protocol. It involves contracting the muscles and tendons around your heel as you lengthen the muscle. An example of this technique involves standing on the edge of a stair and then slowly lowering one or both heels below the edge, while holding on to the banister for balance. You will also be given stretches for the calf and Achilles tendon (see "Stretches for your lower legs," at left) to help prevent tightness that could lead to future injuries.

Special shoes and orthotic devices can make you more comfortable while your injury heals. Soft-backed sneakers or shoes will

---

## Stretches for your lower legs

These exercises stretch the Achilles tendon and the muscles of your calves.

### Standing calf stretch

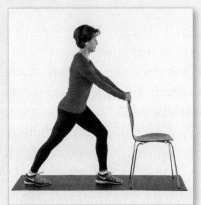

To do this stretch:

- Start by standing up straight. Hold the back of a chair or press your hands against a wall, arms extended at shoulder height.
- Extend your right leg straight back and press the heel into the floor. Allow your left knee to bend as you do so, while keeping that heel grounded on the floor. Feel the stretch in the back of your calf. Hold this position for 10 to 30 seconds. Return to the starting position, then repeat with your left leg. Do the stretch on both sides for a total of two to four times.

### Variation: Seated calf stretch

To do this stretch:

- Sit on the floor with your left leg out straight.
- Bend your right leg in so that the sole of the right foot is pressed against your left upper thigh.
- Lean forward and gently grasp your left foot, pulling it toward you (use a strap if you can't reach your foot).
- Hold the position for 10 to 30 seconds. Repeat on the other side. Do the stretch on both sides for a total of two to four times.

### Standing soleus stretch

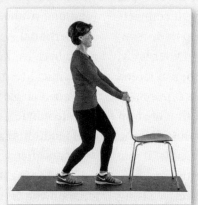

To do this stretch:

- Stand up straight. Hold the back of a chair or press your hands against a wall, arms extended at shoulder height.
- Extend your right leg slightly behind you and press the heel into the floor. Allow your left knee to bend as you do so, while keeping the heel grounded on the floor. Now bend your right knee as much as possible, pressing into your heel until you feel a stretch low in your calf. Hold for 10 to 30 seconds. Return to standing. Do this one to three times more, then repeat the entire sequence with your other leg.

---

prevent any rubbing against the already irritated heel. Shoe inserts called heel lifts raise the heel, moving it away from the back of the shoe to prevent rubbing. Whatever you do, avoid "rocker" shoes, which have a higher forefoot than heel, because they put too much stress on the Achilles tendon.

These treatments should improve Achilles tendinitis, but it can take up to six months to notice a difference.

If you have a tendon tear, your doctor may suggest surgery. In debridement surgery, the surgeon removes the damaged part of the Achilles tendon and then repairs the tear with sutures. Any bone spurs will also be removed during this procedure. If more than half of the Achilles tendon is damaged, the surgeon may remove a piece of tendon from the big toe and use it to shore up the Achilles tendon to prevent it from rupturing again. (This procedure shouldn't affect your ability to walk or run.)

After surgery, you'll need physical therapy for up to a year to fully recover.

# Cellulitis

Cellulitis is a bacterial infection of the skin. Although you can get it in any part of your body, it's most likely to affect your lower legs. Bacteria that normally live on your skin—most commonly *Streptococcus* or *Staphylococcus*—enter your body through a cut, burn, scrape, or surgical wound; a skin condition like eczema or athlete's foot; or another open sore. Increasingly, methicillin-resistant *Staphylococcus aureus* (MRSA) bacteria cause cellulitis. This "superbug" is tough to treat because it's resistant to many commonly used antibiotics. Once inside your body, the bacteria can spread to your lymph nodes and bloodstream, where they can cause a life-threatening infection called sepsis.

Although anyone can get cellulitis, you're more likely to develop this infection if you have one of the following conditions:
- a weakened immune system from a disease, or from chemotherapy or another medical treatment
- a chronic illness such as diabetes
- a skin condition such as eczema or shingles
- obesity.

## ▶ Symptoms of cellulitis
- Swelling and redness of the skin on one leg (the redness may gradually expand)
- Pain and tenderness
- Warmth
- A fever
- Blisters
- Dimpling of the skin

## Diagnosing cellulitis

See a doctor right away if you have a large area of red swollen skin and a fever, or if you notice skin symptoms like these and you have diabetes or a weakened immune system. Cellulitis is a potentially serious condition that needs to be treated as soon as possible. Your doctor should be able to diagnose it just by examining your skin.

## Treating cellulitis

Cellulitis is treated with an oral antibiotic, which you will take for 10 to 14 days. Your symptoms should improve within one to two days, but be sure to finish the entire prescription anyway. Stopping the medicine too soon allows the strongest bacteria to survive, contributing to the development of antibiotic-resistant superbugs—and setting up the possibility that your infection will come roaring back. If you don't feel better or if your symptoms get worse while on oral antibiotics, you may need to be treated with stronger intravenous (IV) antibiotics in a hospital. Severe cases may be treated with IV antibiotics from the start.

When you treat cellulitis early, it usually clears up completely without causing any long-term complications. However, once you've had cellulitis, you are more likely to develop it again. To prevent a future occurrence, keep your skin clean and, if you have any wounds, be sure to properly disinfect and cover them.

# Edema

Edema occurs when fluid becomes trapped in the body's tissues, causing them to swell. The word "edema" comes from the Greek word *oidein*, meaning "to swell." Although edema can occur anywhere in the body, it's most likely to affect the legs, ankles, and feet.

## ▶ Symptoms of edema

- Swelling or puffiness in the legs
- Skin that looks stretched or shiny in the swollen area
- Pitting of the skin when you press on it for five seconds or more
- Difficulty walking due to heaviness or enlargement of the legs

Leg swelling caused by excess fluid buildup is known as peripheral edema.

Many different medical conditions can cause peripheral edema, including

- cardiomyopathy—a disease of the heart muscle that makes it harder for your heart to pump enough blood to your body
- chronic kidney disease or kidney failure—damage to the kidneys that can cause extra fluid and sodium to build up in your bloodstream, leading to swelling
- cirrhosis—scarring of the liver due to excessive alcohol use or diseases such as hepatitis that can cause fluid to build up in the body
- heart failure—an inability of the heart to pump blood effectively, which can make blood pool in the legs and feet
- nephrotic syndrome—kidney disease that causes excessive protein loss in urine, which may in turn lead to a buildup of fluid in the body
- pericarditis—inflammation of the membrane around the heart that can prevent the heart from pumping enough blood, causing blood to build up in the legs
- thrombophlebitis—a condition in which a blood clot (thrombus) forms in one or more superficial veins, usually in the lower leg, causing inflammation of the vein (phlebitis) and preventing normal blood flow
- venous insufficiency—weakening or damage in the leg veins

Edema can occur anywhere in the body, but it's most common in the legs, ankles, and feet. Many conditions, including venous insufficiency and heart failure, can cause it.

that prevents them from pushing enough blood up to the heart, causing blood to leak backward and pool in the legs.

In addition, sitting or standing for long periods of time can produce this symptom, as gravity causes blood to pool in the legs. Too much sodium in your diet can lead to fluid buildup. During pregnancy, extra blood and fluid in the body, along with the additional pressure of the expanding uterus on blood vessels, can make the legs swell. Some medications—including nonsteroidal anti-inflammatory drugs, certain blood pressure medications, steroid drugs, female hormones, and blood pressure medications—may cause edema as a side effect.

## Diagnosing edema

See your doctor if you have symptoms of peripheral edema. If you have symptoms like shortness of breath, trouble breathing, or chest pain, get medical attention right away. These could be signs of fluid buildup in your lungs (pulmonary edema)—which, like edema in the lower legs, can indicate heart failure—or a blood clot in the lungs (pulmonary embolism; see "Deep-vein thrombosis," page 17).

Your doctor may be able to diagnose peripheral edema based on your symptoms and medical history alone, but imaging tests or blood and urine tests are often helpful. Blood tests can reveal heart, liver, or kidney disease. Ultrasound can identify a DVT. And tests like an echocardiogram (which uses high-frequency sound waves to create images of your heart) are helpful for diagnosing a heart condition.

## Treating edema

Some cases of edema may improve on their own if you simply restrict your salt intake and keep your legs propped up on a pillow (ideally above the level of your heart) when you sit or lie down. This

© vchal | Getty Images

encourages blood flow out of your legs and back to your heart. Try not to sit or stand for too long at a time. Wearing compression stockings also prevents blood from pooling in your legs. Limiting sodium and fluid sometimes prevents fluid buildup, especially if you have a condition like heart failure that hinders your heart's pumping ability.

For severe edema, your doctor may prescribe a diuretic, or "water pill," which helps to remove extra fluid and sodium through your urine. You'll also need to treat the cause of edema, which may include therapy to control kidney, liver, or heart disease, or changing medications if one of your drugs causes edema.

# Muscle cramps

The muscles in your legs are made up of bundles of fibers that alternately contract and expand to produce movement. A cramp is a sudden, involuntary contraction (tightening) of one of these muscles, typically in your calf. Cramps can last anywhere from a few seconds to several minutes. They can be mild, or intense enough to wake you out of a sound sleep. A sudden, painful muscle spasm in the leg is called a charley horse, which legend has it is named after baseball player Charlie "Hoss" Radbourn, who reportedly suffered from frequent cramps back in the 1880s.

Sometimes there is no obvious cause for a cramp. Exercise is a common trigger, especially after you've exercised for a long period of time or in the heat. Muscles that are tired or dehydrated become irritated and are more likely to cramp up. A deficiency of electrolytes such as magnesium or potassium in your diet can lead to more frequent cramping, by preventing your muscles from fully relaxing. The risk of a cramp increases during pregnancy, possibly because of circulatory changes and increased stress on the muscles from a growing belly. Age is another fac-

tor, with cramps becoming more frequent in middle age and beyond. Older muscles tire more easily, and they become increasingly sensitive to lower fluid volumes in the body. Cramps can also be a side effect of medicines like statins, which are used to treat high cholesterol.

## Diagnosing muscle cramps

You should be able to treat a cramp on your own, but see a doctor if your cramps are severe, you get them often, or you have other symptoms (like numbness or weakness) along with them. Rarely, cramps can signal a problem with the spine, blood vessels, or liver.

## Treating muscle cramps

Most cramps will go away on their own within a few seconds to minutes. Stretching or massaging the muscle will help it relax. Heat is soothing to tense muscles. Apply a heating pad or warm wet washcloth to help loosen up the muscle.

To avoid leg cramps in the future, drink plenty of fluids before and during exercise. Muscles need fluid to contract and relax properly. Prevent tightness by warming up your leg muscles before you work out with some walking in place or a slow jog. After each workout, stretch out your leg muscles for a few minutes (see "Stretches for your lower legs," page 40). Do another set of stretches before bed if you tend to get cramps while you sleep. For cramps that are especially severe, frequent, or disruptive to sleep, a prescription muscle relaxant like cyclobenzaprine (Flexeril), metaxalone (Skelaxin), or methocarbamol (Robaxin) may help.

# Peripheral artery disease (PAD) and claudication

Peripheral artery disease (PAD) is a narrowing of arteries in the legs (and sometimes the arms)—that is, the body's periphery, or outer areas. Like coronary artery disease, it is caused by the buildup of arterial plaques (deposits of fat, cholesterol, and other substances that collect in your arteries). The blood vessels stiffen as a result and are unable to dilate (widen) enough to deliver sufficient oxygen and nutrients during physical activity.

## ▶ Symptoms of muscle cramps

- Sudden pain and tightness in a muscle, typically in your calf
- A temporary hard lump or twitching under the skin as the muscle contracts

The main symptom of PAD is claudication (pain when you walk or exercise). But in the most serious cases, reduced blood flow can lead to tissue death (gangrene).

PAD is an incredibly common condition, affecting some 8.5 million Americans. Up to one out of every five people over age 60 has it, and only about a quarter of people who are affected realize they are living with PAD.

Having heart disease risk factors such as obesity, high blood pressure and cholesterol, and diabetes raises your odds of developing peripheral artery disease. Smoking is the leading risk factor and the one that increases your chances the most of having serious complications like gangrene in your legs from poor blood flow.

### Diagnosing PAD

Your doctor will examine you, using a stethoscope to listen through the skin over your arteries. A whooshing sound (called a bruit) or weak pulse are signs that blood isn't flowing properly through these vessels. Your primary care doctor can do the initial exam, but for a more comprehensive diagnosis and treatment, you may need to see a vascular surgeon or a cardiologist.

Doctors use a variety of tests to diagnose PAD. The ankle-brachial index compares the blood pressure readings from your upper arm and your ankle;

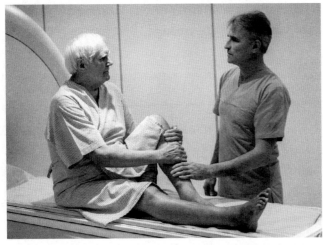

One approach to diagnosing peripheral artery disease involves injecting a contrast dye into your bloodstream, then using imaging to see how the dye (along with your blood) is flowing through your arteries.

## Symptoms of peripheral artery disease (PAD)

- Pain in one or both legs that appears when you walk or climb stairs and disappears when you rest (called intermittent claudication)
- An aching or heaviness in the affected leg
- Weakness or numbness in the leg
- Cold areas on your lower leg or foot
- Sores on your legs or feet that don't heal
- Reddish-blue color to your leg
- Hair loss on your leg
- Shiny skin
- A weak pulse in your legs and feet

blood pressure that is lower in your leg than in your arm may indicate narrowed blood vessels in your legs. Doppler ultrasound uses a small device called a transducer, which emits high-frequency sound waves as a technician rolls it over your leg. The test measures blood flow through the vessels of your legs to identify any narrowing or blockages.

Several tests involve injecting a contrast dye (a substance visible on a particular type of imaging scan) into your bloodstream. Your doctor can watch the dye's progress through your arteries using any of these types of imaging:
- x-rays (in a test called angiography)
- MRI, which uses magnets and radio waves (in a test called magnetic resonance angiography, or MRA)
- CT, which combines x-rays from multiple angles (in a test called computerized tomography angiography, or CTA).

Injecting the dye through a catheter (narrow tube) passed into a blood vessel is a more invasive way to find the source of the problem, but the advantage is that once the narrowed artery is located, the doctor may be able to widen it immediately using medication or by inflating a small balloon inside it.

### Treating PAD

If you have PAD, it's very important to control your vascular disease risk factors. Just as artery narrowing limits blood flow to your legs, it could also disrupt

© skynesher | Getty Images

blood flow to your heart or brain. A piece of plaque can eventually break open and cause a blood clot to form, triggering a heart attack or stroke. Poor blood flow from PAD can lead to the death of tissue in the leg, which could ultimately require amputation.

To prevent PAD—or to avoid complications if you already have it—lose excess weight, quit smoking, and adjust your diet and exercise routine with your doctor's help. If you can't control your cholesterol, blood sugar, and blood pressure with these lifestyle measures alone, ask your doctor whether you need medications to improve your numbers.

For PAD that causes claudication, a few medical procedures are available to open up the blocked area of artery:

- In angioplasty, the doctor threads a catheter through the femoral artery in your groin and advances it to the site of the blockage. A hair-thin wire inserted through this tube allows your surgeon to see inside the artery. Then, a tiny balloon on the end of the catheter is inflated inside the artery to widen it, and sometimes a mesh tube called a stent is put in place to hold the artery open.
- In atherectomy, the doctor uses a catheter with a sharp blade at the end to cut out the blockage.
- In bypass surgery, the doctor places one of your own blood vessels or an artificial graft to direct blood around the blocked artery.

## Peripheral neuropathy

Your peripheral nervous system is an interconnected network of motor and sensory nerves that transmit messages to and from your central nervous system (your brain and spinal cord) and the rest of your body. Signals from motor nerves tell your leg muscles to move so that you can walk and jump. Sensory nerves transmit signals that help you feel the heat of the sun on your bare legs, or the pain from a cut on your shin. Autonomic nerves control functions you don't normally think about, such as breathing, digestion, heart rate, and blood pressure.

Damage to peripheral nerves interrupts or distorts these messages, disrupting whatever function that particular nerve controls. The result is peripheral neuropathy, which causes symptoms like numbness, weakness, pain, or a loss of sensation in the affected area, such as the legs and feet. An estimated 20 million Americans have some type of peripheral neuropathy, although it's difficult to get a precise figure because of the overlap in symptoms with other conditions.

Damage to a single nerve is known as mononeuropathy. When two or more nerves are damaged, doctors refer to it as polyneuropathy.

A number of problems can damage the nerves, including

- diabetes (up to 70% of people with diabetes have some kind of neuropathy, making this the leading cause in the United States)
- an injury from a fall, repetitive use, accident, or sporting activity that compresses, stretches, or damages the nerve
- autoimmune diseases such as Sjögren's syndrome, rheumatoid arthritis, and lupus
- blood vessel problems that reduce blood flow to the peripheral nerves
- kidney and liver diseases
- medications, such as chemotherapy for cancer
- viral infections such as Lyme disease, shingles, chickenpox, Epstein-Barr, HIV, and hepatitis C
- excessive alcohol use
- exposure to chemical toxins such as acrylamide, ethylene glycol (antifreeze), dioxins, lead, or mercury
- tumors that press on nerves
- B vitamin deficiencies
- hereditary disorders such as Charcot-Marie-Tooth disease.

▷ **Symptoms of peripheral neuropathy**
- Numbness, tingling, or a pins-and-needles sensation in your feet and legs
- Burning, sharp, stabbing, electric, or throbbing pain
- Muscle weakness
- Extreme sensitivity to touch
- Muscle cramps or twitches
- Difficulty with balance and coordination

## Diagnosing peripheral neuropathy

Your doctor will ask about your medical history, including what medical conditions, injuries, or medicines might have caused nerve damage. These questions will most likely be followed by a neurological exam in which the doctor checks your muscle strength, reflexes, balance, coordination, and the sensation in your legs and feet.

Blood tests are helpful in detecting an autoimmune disease, diabetes, or a vitamin deficiency. A CT or MRI scan may be done to look for an injury such as a herniated disc or a tumor that is putting pressure on a nerve. Your doctor might also perform nerve conduction velocity and electromyography tests, which measure nerve strength and speed and detect the electrical activity in your muscles to identify a potential nerve problem (see "Nerve studies," page 25). Sometimes the diagnosis requires a nerve biopsy, in which the doctor removes a small piece of a sensory nerve from your lower leg and sends it to a lab to check for any problems. A skin biopsy (removal of a small piece of skin for testing) can detect problems with nerve fibers in the skin.

## Treating peripheral neuropathy

The primary goal of treatment is to control the underlying condition that is causing the nerve damage. That could entail taking medications for diabetes or an autoimmune disease, or removing a tumor or spinal disc that's putting pressure on a nerve. The hope is that addressing the problem will relieve the pain, numbness, and tingling.

In addition, your doctor may recommend a drug to relieve symptoms. Drugs that are used to treat peripheral neuropathy include the following:

- Over-the-counter pain relievers—either acetaminophen (Tylenol) or nonsteroidal anti-inflammatory drugs such as aspirin, ibuprofen, or naproxen—may work for mild nerve pain.
- Tricyclic antidepressants, such as amitriptyline (Elavil) or nortriptyline (Pamelor), and serotonin-norepinephrine reuptake inhibitors (SNRIs), such as duloxetine (Cymbalta), can alter the brain signals that cause you to feel pain.
- Antiseizure drugs such as gabapentin (Neurontin) and pregabalin (Lyrica) can help relieve nerve pain.
- Topical pain relievers, such as patches or creams containing lidocaine or capsaicin, can block the sensation of pain in the area where you apply them.
- Opioid medications may be tried if other treatments haven't worked. Because of the risk of dependence and side effects, however, these drugs should be used sparingly and only under the close supervision of a doctor.

A noninvasive treatment called transcutaneous electrical nerve stimulation (TENS) can be helpful for peripheral neuropathy, especially when diabetes is the cause. You place electrodes attached to a battery-operated unit onto your skin for about 30 minutes a day. The electrodes emit a gentle current, which is believed to work by interfering with the transmission of pain signals to the brain and stimulating the release of pain-relieving chemicals in the body. Although research hasn't confirmed that TENS is effective for peripheral neuropathy, it is unlikely to cause side effects other than mild skin irritation where the electrodes are placed.

If a nerve is compressed—for example, by a herniated spinal disc or a tumor—surgery may be performed to release the nerve.

# Pseudoclaudication (lumbar spine stenosis)

Like claudication (see "Peripheral artery disease and claudication," page 43), pseudoclaudication causes pain in the legs while walking, but for different reasons. Rather than being caused by poor blood flow, pseudoclaudication results from nerve compression in the spine. It is a symptom of spinal stenosis, a narrowing of the spinal canal—the hollow space through which the spinal cord runs as it extends down the back. As the spinal canal narrows, it compresses the nerve roots that branch off the spinal cord. The narrowing is often due to osteoarthritis (which may lead to the growth of bone spurs) or a bulging disc. Degenerated discs and bone spurs can put pressure on nerves of the spine, causing symptoms like pain, numbness, and weakness. If spinal stenosis affects the nerves that control feeling and movement in your lower legs, that's where you will feel the symptoms.

## ▶ Symptoms of pseudoclaudication

- Pain in your legs that gets worse when you stand or walk, and improves when you sit down or bend forward
- Numbness, tingling, and weakness in the legs
- Lower back pain
- Loss of control over your bowels or bladder (rarely)
- Difficulty with sexual function

Because osteoarthritis is so often the cause, pseudoclaudication is more common in older adults. Most people over age 60 will have at least some degree of spinal stenosis. In people ages 50 and younger, the cause is likely congenital spinal stenosis—that is, a narrowing that was present at birth.

### Diagnosing pseudoclaudication

Your doctor will ask about your symptoms and examine your back and legs, as well as do a thorough neurologic exam to rule out other conditions. He or she may also use various types of imaging to help pinpoint a diagnosis:

- An MRI or CT scan may be used to get more detailed images of the spinal cord and confirm that you have spinal stenosis.
- An x-ray can reveal bone spurs, damage to the discs, and narrowing of your spine.
- A myelogram, in which the doctor injects a contrast dye into the spine before performing an x-ray or CT scan, will show the nerves of your spine more clearly than either type of imaging alone.

In addition, two tests—electromyography and nerve conduction studies—can evaluate the speed and strength of nerve impulses and determine how well your nerves are signaling the muscles of your legs (see "Nerve studies," page 25).

### Treating pseudoclaudication

Treatment often starts with physical therapy exercises to strengthen the muscles of your legs and belly, and stretches to relieve pain. The purpose is to open up the spinal canal, although it may not help much for spinal stenosis. An over-the-counter anti-inflammatory pain reliever such as aspirin, ibuprofen, or naproxen can help bring down inflammation and relieve pain in the spine and legs. Corticosteroid injections into the spine (called epidural injections) can also reduce swelling and pain, but they carry a small risk of infection or bleeding and they aren't always effective. Also, you shouldn't have more than a few injections a year.

If your symptoms interfere with your daily life, are severe, or continue to worsen with treatment, you may want to consider a surgery called decompression laminectomy. During this procedure, the surgeon removes any bone spurs, along with the roof (lamina) of one or more vertebrae, to create more space for your spinal nerves. This procedure can be done as open surgery or laparoscopically (using miniature tools inserted through smaller incisions). A spinal fusion, which connects or fuses two or more vertebrae to stabilize your spine, may be done at the same time.

## Restless legs syndrome (RLS)

A creepy, crawly sensation in your legs at night that prevents you from falling asleep could be restless legs syndrome (RLS), also known as Willis-Ekbom disease. Doctors don't know what causes these strange sensations, but they may stem from an imbalance of the brain chemical dopamine, which helps to control muscle movement.

Up to 10% of Americans have this condition. Although RLS can affect people of both genders and all ages, it is more common in women, especially during pregnancy. The frequency also increases with age.

### Diagnosing RLS

Your doctor will ask about your symptoms. The hallmark criterion for a diagnosis of RLS is a crawling or other sensation in your legs at night that makes you want to move your legs, and which improves when you walk or stretch. You may also have a neurological exam and blood tests to rule out other possible causes for your symptoms, such as nerve damage or an iron deficiency.

### Treating RLS

Simple, nonmedical measures may be enough to relieve RLS and help you sleep through the night. Take a warm bath and massage your lower legs before bedtime to relax your muscles. You can also place a heating pad or ice pack on your legs. (Always place a cloth or towel between the ice pack and your skin, to avoid damaging the skin.) Exercise daily, but do it early in the day to avoid disrupting your sleep even more. Try to get to bed early each night, and keep your bedroom comfortably dark and cool to promote better sleep. Avoid caffeine and alcohol, especially before bed. Both can worsen RLS symptoms. If you're low on iron, your doctor might suggest taking a supplement.

In addition, the FDA has recently cleared a couple of devices to treat RLS. One is a foot wrap called Restiffic that goes around the middle of your foot. It relieves RLS symptoms by putting gentle pressure on muscles in the bottom of your foot. The other device, called Relaxis, is a vibrating pad that you place under your lower legs for about 30 minutes at a time. Studies suggest that Relaxis improves the ability to sleep, but the evidence is not compelling for either device. Both devices are available only with a prescription from your doctor. Restiffic costs about $200, while Relaxis costs about $700, and neither is typically covered by insurance.

The following medicines, primarily used for other conditions, can also help with RLS:

- Parkinson's drugs such as pramipexole (Mirapex), ropinirole (Requip), and rotigotine (Neupro) ease RLS symptoms by increasing dopamine levels in the brain.
- Antiseizure drugs like gabapentin, gabapentin enacarbil (Horizant), and pregabalin may help with RLS symptoms.
- Muscle relaxants like clonazepam (Klonopin) can

help you fall asleep, although they don't treat the abnormal leg sensations.

These drugs can cause side effects, including daytime drowsiness and dizziness. Use them only when necessary and under the direction of your doctor.

# Shin splints

Your shin bone (tibia) runs down the front of your lower leg, from your knee to your ankle. The term "shin splints" refers to pain and inflammation of your tibia and its associated muscles and tendons, caused by overworking this region. You are most likely to get shin splints if you increase your activity level; for example, if you switch from a daily 30-minute walk to an hour walk, or you add more hills to your runs. Runners face the highest risk for shin splints, followed by dancers and military recruits. Running or dancing on a hard surface like concrete increases the risk for shin splints.

You're more likely to develop this problem if you have flat feet, because without the proper arches, your feet don't provide adequate shock absorption for your lower legs. Wearing inappropriate shoes or worn-out sneakers increases your likelihood of developing this condition.

## Diagnosing shin splints

Your doctor will ask about your symptoms and examine your lower legs. An x-ray, MRI, or other imaging test can help rule out conditions with similar symptoms, such as tendinitis or a stress fracture in your tibia.

## Treating shin splints

Because overuse is the main cause of shin splints, rest is often the solution. Avoid the activity that caused your pain. If you are a frequent walker or jogger, substitute a non-impact activity such as swimming or bike riding. To bring down swelling and reduce pain, hold an ice pack to your shin for about 20 minutes at a time, several times a day. An over-the-counter anti-inflammatory pain reliever such as aspirin, ibuprofen, or naproxen may also help with both swelling and pain.

Stretch your lower leg muscles a few times a day

---

▶ **Symptoms of restless legs syndrome (RLS)**

- A crawling, throbbing, creeping, aching, tingling, or other abnormal sensation in your legs, often occurring at night, that is relieved by movements like walking or stretching
- An urgent need to move your legs

- Throbbing, dull, or sharp pain in the front of your lower legs
- Pain that gets worse when you exercise

to keep your muscles limber. Wear good, supportive shoes with adequate cushioning throughout the day to reduce the stress on your shins. (If you're a runner, see "How to find the right running shoes," page 22.) Orthotic shoe inserts can help realign your foot and ankle and take pressure off your shins. These inserts may be particularly useful if you have flat feet, or if you frequently get shin splints.

Shin splints can take up to six months to heal. Don't return to the activity that caused them until you've been pain-free for at least two weeks, and then only gradually ease back into your program. Rushing back into your sport or activity could lead to another injury.

# Skin ulcers (leg ulcers)

A skin ulcer is a medical term for a sore or opening in the skin. Ulcers caused by an injury are typically one-time occurrences. However, when they result from an underlying medical problem, these sores can be slow to heal, putting you at risk for infections if bacteria or other germs make their way into your body through the opening. You can also develop pressure sores if you are bedridden; in the lower legs, these may occur on the heels.

By far the most common cause of leg ulcers is chronic venous insufficiency (improper functioning of the valves in leg veins), which is responsible for about 80% of all leg ulcers. As discussed earlier (see "Leg anatomy: An overview," page 2), veins are the blood vessels that carry oxygen-depleted blood from your legs back up to your heart. However, aging and inactivity can cause the one-way valves in leg veins to malfunction, so that blood pools in the legs rather than continuing to move back up toward the heart. You're more likely to develop this condition after having deep-vein thrombosis (see page 17),

which can damage the valves in your veins. If you don't treat chronic venous insufficiency, blood can eventually spill over into the tiny capillaries of your legs and quickly overwhelm them to the point where they burst open. The broken blood vessels weaken and damage the skin above them, producing an open sore.

While problems with veins are the most common cause of leg ulcers, poor blood flow in the arteries of the legs can also cause them. A lack of blood flow compromises the quality of the skin and its ability to withstand minor injuries and heal properly. Other possible causes include

- diabetes, due to a combination of poor blood flow (from blood vessel damage) and nerve damage (which prevents people from feeling injuries when they occur); however, ulcers from diabetes are more likely to form on the feet than on the legs
- kidney failure—in rare cases, from calcium buildup in the small blood vessels that deprives the skin of oxygen and nutrients
- rheumatoid arthritis and other inflammatory diseases—sometimes because of inflammation in blood vessels supplying the skin, sometimes because of infection, and other times because of venous insufficiency
- cellulitis (see page 41)
- an injury that breaks the skin and leaves a sore or opening
- lying down for long periods of time, such as following surgery.

## Diagnosing leg ulcers

For a thorough diagnosis and treatment, you may need to see a wound specialist, vascular surgeon, or both. To diagnose venous insufficiency, your doctor

▶ **Symptoms of leg ulcers**

- One or more open sores on the leg
- Red, brown, or purple skin (a sign that blood has pooled beneath the skin)
- Dry, scaly skin around the ulcer
- Swelling of the leg

may use a test called a vascular ultrasound. A transducer releases sound waves, which bounce off of blood vessels and other structures in your leg to produce an image on a monitor.

### Treating leg ulcers

The goal in treating skin ulcers is to encourage wound healing and prevent infection. To these ends, your doctor may prescribe special wound dressings and antibiotics. You will need to keep the dressing clean and dry. Change it as often as your doctor recommends. Compression, which is accomplished by wearing special stockings or wrapping a bandage around the leg, can help bring down swelling.

Chronic venous insufficiency is treated with regular exercise and loss of excess weight. Try to avoid sitting or standing for long periods of time. Every few minutes, get up and walk to encourage blood flow in your legs. Wearing compression stockings can also help keep blood flowing in the right direction.

Ulcers are notoriously slow to heal. It may take four months or longer for the wound to completely clear up. Once it has healed, you will need to take good care of your legs, and possibly continue to wear compression stockings to prevent another ulcer from forming. Many people find off-the-shelf compression stockings uncomfortable; however, a doctor can help make sure you have the correct size with the proper amount of compression.

It's important to carefully clean and inspect the skin of your legs and feet every day, especially if you have diabetes. Diabetic nerve damage can prevent you from feeling an injury if one occurs. Wash your legs and feet with a mild soap and warm water, then gently pat them dry. Apply moisturizer to your skin to prevent cracks that can open up into sores.

# Varicose veins

Veins are the networks of blood vessels that carry blood from your legs back to your heart. From the legs to the heart is a long trip that requires blood to flow against the downward pull of gravity. Along with the leg muscles, which squeeze the veins to push blood upward, the leg veins come equipped with one-way valves to help keep blood flowing in the right direction. If these valves malfunction or if they are damaged, blood can pool inside the veins and cause them to swell. Phlebitis is the term used to describe an inflamed vein.

Varicose veins are swollen veins close to the surface of the skin—generally in the lower leg, although they can occur in the upper leg, too. Backed-up blood stretches the walls of these veins, turning them thick and ropey. As the enlarged veins try to squeeze into the same space they've always inhabited, they twist up. For many people, varicose veins are primarily a cosmetic issue, but they can cause pain, too—particularly after you've been sitting or standing for a long time. Sometimes a blood clot forms in a varicose vein or another surface vein—a painful and annoying but rarely serious condition called superficial thrombophlebitis.

Twice as many women develop varicose veins as men, in part because of hormonal changes that occur during life transitions such as pregnancy and menopause. Aging itself can cause wear-and-tear on the veins that eventually makes their walls and valves weaken. Being overweight puts added pressure on these veins.

### Diagnosing varicose veins

Although your primary care doctor can make the initial diagnosis based on your symptoms and the appearance of veins in your legs, you may need to see a vascular specialist, dermatologist, or plastic surgeon if the diagnosis is unclear. Doppler ultrasound is a test commonly used to diagnose varicose veins. It uses sound waves to create images of the veins, which can help your doctor identify weak veins and blockages in blood flow. Less commonly, your doctor might order a test called a venogram, in which a dye is injected into a vein, so it will show up more clearly on an x-ray image.

> ### ▶ Symptoms of varicose veins
>
> - Thick, ropey blue or purple veins just under the surface of the skin
> - Aching, throbbing, or heaviness in your legs
> - Itching in your lower legs and ankles

## Treating varicose veins

Varicose veins are typically more annoying than harmful. If they don't bother you or cause symptoms, you don't have to do anything to treat them. You can bring down swelling with the following strategies:

- Stand up and walk around every hour or so throughout the day to keep the blood flowing in your legs.

- Elevate your legs above the level of your heart—for example, by propping them on a pillow—three or four times a day.

- Lose weight if you are overweight or obese, to take pressure off your veins.

- Don't wear leggings or other tight pants that could inhibit the blood flow in your legs.

- Wear compression stockings, which are designed to squeeze the veins in a way that keeps blood moving upward and prevents it from pooling in your legs. You can buy these stockings over the counter at a drugstore. If you find the store-bought stockings too uncomfortable, have some custom-fit for you with a prescription from your doctor.

Several medical procedures treat varicose veins, either by sealing off or removing them. Once a vein is closed or removed, the blood flow simply reroutes around it.

**Sclerotherapy.** This is the most common treatment for varicose veins. The doctor injects a chemical into the vein, which irritates and scars it to the point where the vein eventually closes. This procedure is

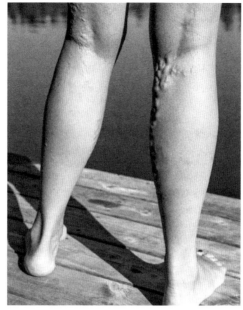

Varicose veins are primarily a cosmetic issue, but sometimes they can cause pain—particularly after you've been sitting or standing for a long time.

typically done once every four to six weeks until the affected veins have faded away.

**Thermal ablation therapy.** The doctor makes a small cut in the skin and places a thin tube called a catheter inside the vein. Laser or radiofrequency energy passed through the catheter heats and seals off the vein.

**Ambulatory phlebectomy.** The doctor makes small cuts in the skin and uses special hooks to pull the veins out of your legs. This procedure can remove varicose veins that are close to the surface.

**Vein stripping and ligation.** This procedure ties off and removes the damaged veins through small openings in the skin. It is typically reserved for severe varicose veins.

## Care for your legs, protect your health

The conditions highlighted in this report illustrate the relationship between your leg health and overall health. When something is wrong with your legs—a nagging ache, muscle weakness, swelling, or numbness—it could signal a more serious problem that needs your attention. Give just as much care and concern to your legs as you would to your heart, lungs, brain, and other vital organs. Your legs are key to maintaining your independence as you age. The better you care for them, the more likely they'll be able to support you for the rest of your life. ▼

# Resources

## Organizations

**American Academy of Orthopaedic Surgeons (AAOS)**
9400 W. Higgins Road
Rosemont, IL 60018
800-626-6726 (toll-free)
https://orthoinfo.aaos.org

The American Academy of Orthopaedic Surgeons is a national organization of orthopedic specialists. The AAOS has a comprehensive website, called OrthoInfo, filled with informative articles about arthritis, fractures, tendon and muscle injuries, and other conditions affecting the musculoskeletal system.

**American College of Rheumatology (ACR)**
2200 Lake Blvd. NE
Atlanta, GA 30319
404-633-3777
www.rheumatology.org

This website for rheumatology professionals includes a consumer-friendly section, complete with overviews of rheumatic diseases such as arthritis. It includes information on what to do when you're newly diagnosed, how to manage your medications, and how to live better with these conditions.

**American Orthopaedic Society for Sports Medicine (AOSSM)**
9400 W. Higgins Road, Suite 300
Rosemont, IL 60018
877-321-3500 (toll-free)
www.sportsmed.org

This organization of sports medicine professionals offers a patient-focused newsletter as well as an online directory of specialists on its website. You'll also find tip sheets and resources to help prevent sports injuries in both children and adults.

**American Physical Therapy Association**
1111 N. Fairfax St.
Alexandria, VA 22314
800-999-2782 (toll-free)
www.apta.org

This professional organization represents more than 100,000 physical therapists around the country. On its consumer website, www.moveforwardpt.com, you can read patient stories and find a physical therapist in your area.

**Arthritis Foundation**
1355 Peachtree St. NE, 6th Floor
Atlanta, GA 30309
404-872-7100
844-571-HELP (toll-free)
www.arthritis.org

The website of this national nonprofit organization has educational materials on arthritis, joint surgery, pain control, and standard and complementary therapies, as well as exercise videos and a directory of local offices and events. Local chapters may offer joint-health exercise classes, including water-based classes.

**National Institute of Arthritis and Musculoskeletal and Skin Diseases (NIAMS)**
1 AMS Circle
Bethesda, MD 20892
877-226-4267 (toll-free)
www.niams.nih.gov

This division of the National Institutes of Health deals with arthritis and other diseases of the musculoskeletal system. Its website includes a variety of informational resources.

## Publications from Harvard Medical School

The following Special Health Reports and Online Guides from Harvard Medical School go into greater detail on various topics mentioned in this report. You can order them by going to www.health.harvard.edu or calling 877-649-9457 (toll-free).

**Finding Relief for Sciatica** (2018). This online-only guide explains the causes of and treatments for sciatica, including medications, surgery, and physical therapy. Includes home remedies and the importance of good posture and getting enough sleep.

**Healthy Feet: Preventing and treating common foot problems** (2018). This Special Health Report covers 30 different problems that can affect your feet, from bunions to toenail fungus. It includes a Special Section on keeping your feet healthy.

**The Joint Pain Relief Workout: Healing exercises for your shoulders, hips, knees, and ankles** (2018). The expert-designed workouts in this report are intended to strengthen the muscles that support your joints, increase flexibility, and improve range of motion. Done regularly, these exercises can ease your pain, improve mobility, and help prevent injury.

**Knees and Hips: A troubleshooting guide to knee and hip pain** (2018). This Special Health Report describes the most common knee and hip problems and the best treatments for them. A Special Section provides in-depth information on joint replacement.

**Living Well with Osteoarthritis: A guide to keeping your joints healthy** (2019). Osteoarthritis—the most common type of arthritis—can interfere with your quality of life. This Special Health Report covers the many ways you can protect your joints, reduce discomfort, and improve mobility.

**Stretching: 35 stretches to improve flexibility and reduce pain** (2017). Several of the stretches illustrated in *Healing Leg Pain* were drawn from *Stretching*. This Special Health Report includes stretches that can help you increase your flexibility, improve your balance, and reduce pain and stiffness.

**Total Hip Replacement: What you need to know about getting a new joint** (2018). This online-only guide walks you through the process of deciding if a hip replacement is right for you, sorting through the various options, and handling rehab.

**Total Knee Replacement: What you need to know about getting a new joint** (2018). This online-only guide helps you sort through the options and prepare for surgery.